RESPONDING TO THE **MASS CASUALTY** INCIDENT: A Guide for EMS Personnel

RESPONDING TO THE **MASS CASUALTY** INCIDENT: A Guide for EMS Personnel

Alexander M. Butman, EMSI
Executive Director, Emergency Training
Adjunct Professor of Emergency Medical Services,
Central Connecticut State College,
New Britain, Connecticut

EMERGENCY TRAINING
miller landing building 200
150 north miller road, akron, ohio 44313

Grateful acknowledgment is made to:

- The members of the Florida Chapter of The American College of Emergency Physicians, its staff, and especially Executive Director Garry L. Briese. Their three annual conferences—*Disasters: Problems and Solutions in Their Management*—have made a major contribution to this book.

- The men and women of the Weston Emergency Medical Services and the many other services and individuals from the Southwestern Connecticut Emergency Medical Services Region who were involved in the Mass Casualty Program. Their insights, knowledge, and hard work throughout the planning, preparation, and execution of numerous drills and exercises were an essential part of the experience necessary in putting together this text.

Printed in the United States of America

ISBN 0-940432-02-1

This book is for Ian and Evan

Contents

Preface

The validation of medical knowledge occurs through a long and complicated chain of events — from controlled experiments in a single location to widespread testing involving many independent practitioners and institutions. Soon afterward, personal validation commences as individual physicians, Emergency Departments, and Emergency Medical Services employ the new device or technique. These individuals and organizations can then see the results firsthand and determine whether or not they match the reported results.*

In the normal delivery of patient care we daily validate, alter, and revalidate our practices based upon our *real experience* and our *deductive ability*. By contrast, in the area of Mass Casualty Patient Care, there is no daily method of validation. The extension of everyday EMS practices into mass casualty situations produces many invalid conclusions.

It is also apparent that there is virtually no way of becoming an expert through vast experience at actual incidents. Even the most seasoned veterans rarely have had experience with more than 2 or 3 Mass Casualty Incidents (MCIs). (I have only met one person who has been at 5.) Futhermore, "controlled" experimentation cannot be attempted during an actual incident, and time pressures do not allow for careful record keeping. Lastly, the sharing of detailed information has been guarded and limited. (An open forum would help us save lives, but such a forum is unrealistic in our litigious society.)

Rare as it is, personal experience at even *several* incidents does not assure one of a good overview of this complex subject. The experience potential for the individual is too small, and the scope is too narrow. Generalizing from one or even 2 MCI' s can

*For example, when logrolling of patients with possible spine injury in order to place them on a long board was first introduced, my experience with it was poor. I observed that the technique, regardless of how carefully done, appeared to cause a major relocation of the spine, particularly in the lumbar and cervical areas. Since such a relocation is contraindicated, we stopped using the technique. My initial observations were easily supported, both deductively and empirically. A rudimentary knowledge of anatomy allows us to *deduce* that when the patient is rolled from his back to his side, the spine will relocate. The outermost measure of the shoulders and hips is greater than that at the waist. Therefore, when rolled, the patient sags at the waist so that the median line of the pelvis and shoulder girdle are no longer perpendicular to the spine. This causes a relocation of the lumbar spine. Any major relocation in the lower spine (lumbar or sacral) has an associated relocation in the cervical spine. This hypothesis can also be verified *empirically*. When we logrolled a healthy volunteer, we *saw* the change. An X ray of the volunteer showed the misalignment and potential stress. Finally, when I had my associates logroll me, I *felt* my spine relocate.

easily result in misleading conclusions. A sample of one or 2 is too sensitive both to local conditions and to peculiarities related to the mechanism of those incidents. For example, if one generalizes one's experience from a tornado, one can come up with a good plan for *tornadoes in that region*. The plan might or might not be valid for tornadoes in other places, and it might or might not be valid for other types of incidents produced by other causes.

The net result, therefore, is that those who plan for MCIs have usually had neither relevant experience nor adequate literature to rely on. Most of the available literature is either limited to a single aspect (equipment, communication, etc.) or recounts a single incident.

Since daily EMS experience does not provide a projectable measure of potential success or failure in the area of Mass Casualty Patient Care, and since the normal methods of adjusting and validating are not possible, an alternative process had to be devised:

1. The material in this book was based upon an analysis of a wide range of different MCIs. Some involved firsthand experience, but *most* were analyzed from primary and secondary reports. The major premises came from an examination of these incidents. The individual premises and the overall plan were then projected back against the information surrounding each incident to see if they held up. They either did, or were adjusted until all premises stood up to examination across all incidents included. Once the material no longer needed adjustment when it was projected across each incident, we were assured of its reliability. Furthermore, as new incidents not included in our examination occurred, we projected the material over the events at these MCIs, and found that it continued to hold up without alteration.

2. Over the last 3 years the major premises and general plan in this book have been exposed to a vast audience of personnel experienced in actual mass casualty responses and in EMS preplanning and training. Although some details led to differences of opinion, ("In our area we handle the problem by . . . instead of by . . .") *no major premise was consistently or even regularly challenged as incorrect or fallacious*—except one. At almost every presentation, the criteria for triage were challenged by a *small* number of participants who could not accept the concept of the catastrophically injured being relegated to second priority. However, the majority agreed that, although this is contrary to daily EMS practice and contrary to our emotional preset, it is an essential practice if we are to focus on *all* urgent patients' needs rather than on any one individual's. (This concept is, in fact, essential to the very purpose of mass casualty triage: the saving of the most lives possible.)

Finally, we reached a point in the development of the material when no questions or challenges arose from a wide range of participants *that had not already been heard and were not included or answered.* *

3. Everyone I have ever met who has seen a Mass Casualty Incident *and* has observed a mass casualty drill or practice exercise, agrees that no *real* response has ever been as bad as the "responses" observed at disaster drills. (I've been an observer and/or an umpire at a large number of these exercises, most of which can best be characterized as either total chaos or worse. In fact, most are so bad that one would imagine some element in the responders was *attempting* to produce confusion and anarchy.) We concluded that, since actual responses are better than exercises, if our system worked to answer the problems at exercises it would work to answer the problems at incidents. In a large number of cases where exercises were chaotic and resulted in poor mock care, responders were then trained in the basic material covered in this book and an ensuing exercise was held. In *each* instance the proper resources arrived and patient care followed previously determined criteria for triage. Regardless of the various levels of leadership, command and order were maintained at all times in the field, and no overall failures in treatment, transportation, use of resources or communication prevailed. Some individual lapses did occur—either as exceptions (related to an individual responder's poor judgment) or as a result of temporary failure of equipment or sequence. In each case, however, such failures were recognized rapidly and were rectified by those in command within a reasonable time. The ultimate result was that any major shortcoming was corrected either before it had any effect, or while its effect was still limited to very few patients. Observable results have been the same even when the material has been taught to responders by persons other than myself or my associates.

As each Mass Casualty Incident occurs there are new lessons to be learned. Like most major areas of EMS, MCIs present an endless avenue for study and learning. The general principles, the common needs and problems, and the general framework of an ef-

*On one other occasion the need for tagging was challenged on the basis of time spent. Any argument against tagging and recording brief patient data mistakes haste for speed. *Less* time is involved in tagging and recording than in reconstructing "lost" information and re-evaluating people because no short patient record was established. In daily EMS — when time is of the essence — ambulance and ED charting can be done after the fact, with all pertinent information exchanged orally. However, in a Mass Casualty Incident, patient care is neither continuous, nor does it permit continuity of personnel. Therefore, the tags and short record are essential: they represent the only link for continuity of care.

fective response, however, do not change materially—they change only in translation and adaptation to the specific details of each incident.

The training of responders in the plan presented in this book, and the application of this training at a variety of ensuing incidents, will, within the limits that one can gather information surrounding a Mass Casualty Incident, prove whether or not the plan can withstand the test of wide MCI application. We will learn how to improve, enlarge and modify the material so that our knowledge and experience will grow.

It is our hope that when a second study of the quality of EMS in disasters is made, it will show that patients *were* afforded the same levels and quality of stabilization as are provided in daily care; that the EMS response effectively reduced morbidity and mortality; and that in the midst of the chaos of a disaster this plan provided a meaningful order that helped to save the greatest possible number of lives.

Chapter 1

MASS CASUALTY: MYTH AND REALITY

The State of the Art

Before going through a detailed consideration of the elements of a *Mass Casualty Incident* (MCI) and the EMS response, it is important to correct certain common misconceptions.

There is probably no subject in the EMS field that is as little understood and, therefore, as poorly handled as mass casualty. In most cases, there is neither preplanning nor training; or, even worse, there is a plan that starts with incorrect assumptions and then develops invalidly. Both instances result in a response that is unrealistic and inadequate. As will be demonstrated, there is a vast difference between the common preconceptions of what *will* occur, and what actually *does* occur in a Mass Casualty Incident.

A COMMUNITY'S PRECONCEPTIONS

In discussions of their community's "mass casualty plan," reliable, highly experienced emergency executives, involved in the daily delivery of emergency medical services, made what can only be described as preposterous statements:

> "We can get 15 ambulances to our community in 10 minutes."
>
> "Through mutual aid we can get 50 additional EMTs there in another 10 to 15 minutes."
>
> "If necessary, I can rapidly get even more ambulances."
>
> "It will be tight, but we can handle 45—even 50 patients in our Emergency Department if we have to."
>
> "We have a whole floor that's unused, so we can handle 100 extra patients at any time if we have 15 minutes' warning. Beds aren't a problem for us."
>
> "I can get a medical team out to the site in 10 minutes."

When any statement was challenged, heated debate ensued. The discussion became more and more emotional—even testy. The implication was that time was being wasted by a compulsion to correct "minor" points.

> "Okay, so it could take 12 minutes, not 10; and one of the 10 ambulances won't be available."
>
> "Maybe I was overly enthusiastic! Fifty is a bit high. But we can handle 40 patients without any problem. Let's get on with it. It's getting late."

Since the participants had adjusted their estimates to a more conservative position, it might have seemed unreasonable to continue challenging these "minor" details. After all, by how much could they be wrong? Two percent? Five percent? Even 10 percent? What everyone failed to grasp was the *compounding* effect of so many interacting errors.

Then came the summation: "If we can get 14 ambulances there in 12 minutes, and each can handle 2 patients at a time . . . and it's 10 minutes to the hospital, we can clear 80 patients from any location within 50 to 60 minutes of the first call." Furthermore, it was concluded that the hospital facilities could easily handle this load.

At our next meeting, we were to discuss what levels of treatment and types of triage were to be performed at each location. The estimated time frames and capacities, now carved in stone, would form the basis upon which we would build the rest of the plan. There were only two things wrong. First, at almost every step the estimates were incorrect. Second, response-time problems and additional factors not apparent to people without experience in mass casualty were not considered.

Because the conclusions were based upon an item-by-item approach, none of the participants was willing to check the sum totals of the final plan against the actual resources of their community. But the plan and the resources simply didn't match, and the differences were sizable enough to make the plan an unworkable piece of fiction.

A decision was made to test some of the items. First, a timed trial run was set up at 2 AM on a night when the weather was clear. This would determine optimum times, since there was no rain, snow, or traffic to contend with. From the moment of notification, it took the dispatcher over 6 minutes to alert all 15 ambulances. Two ambulances were at the site in under 4 minutes; another 2 in under 10. *None* of the remaining 11 were there in under 10 minutes; and the last one arrived 28 minutes from the time the dispatcher had called. Ensuing tests proved:

1. It took 40 minutes to get 22 extra EMTs. (The preconceived number of 50 EMTs was only readily available at night and Sundays.)
2. Only 4 other ambulances (beyond the first 15) could respond in a reasonable time.
3. The Emergency Department could handle only 22 patients at a time, and could rotate this load only every 15 to 20 minutes.
4. Although the hospital could *house* 100 patients with a few minutes' notice, it could not *care* for them. Availability of Operating Rooms, instruments, autoclaving time, and other stabilization and treatment facilities had been overlooked.

Almost everything would take twice as long as was expected; resources and capacities were about half of what was projected; and the ultimate abilities had been overestimated 2- or 3-fold. Actually, the community could handle only 40 serious patients within the time frames that must be assumed.

CONCLUSIONS

The same inaccuracies were found in the plans of most of the other communities we worked with. In fact, of 27 communities, only 2 mass casualty plans were accurate to within 30 percent of the actual capabilities.

More devastating is the fact that the majority of the plans studied do not reflect an understanding of the underlying problems inherent in a Mass Casualty Incident. "Enlargement" plans (doing more and doing it faster)—designed to provide the same care in the same manner as the usual daily delivery of EMS—simply don't work. This is because, *by definition,* there will not be enough time to obtain the necessary resources to provide emergency medical care in the usual way. This inevitably results in inappropriate care: some patients receive all of the available care; others receive very little or none at all. Time and time again the catastrophically injured, who have almost no chance of survival, are provided with heroic resuscitation efforts and are transported by the first crews, leaving little or no personnel and equipment in the field. This situation is commonplace, not the exception.

Our experiences with Mass Casualty Incidents, and our study of others, clearly indicate that the emergency medical services supplied are generally inadequate. In fact, they are usually considerably poorer than the accepted daily minimum standards of emergency care, and could best be described as erratic and chaotic.

It is interesting to note that estimates of fire equipment and manpower were generally realistic. In almost every instance, the fire department could deliver what they said they would. The same was found true of rescue units. The estimates of police manpower and response times were also accurate. However, when compared with experience at actual incidents, mass casualty plans consistently underestimated the number of police officers needed.

Ohio State University Study

In December of 1977, an in-depth study of Mass Casualty Incidents was published that crystallized these shortcomings. *The Delivery of Emergency Medical Services in Disasters* is a study by the Disaster Research Center of the Department of Sociology, The Ohio State University, Columbus, Ohio. The study included field work done in 44 communities located in 17 states, Washington, D.C., and the U.S. Virgin Islands. The research covered localities from small towns to metropolitan areas and included communities with a wide range of EMS development, from very rudimentary capabilities to complex and well-established systems. The study encompassed 29 disasters:

Floods—Wilkes-Barre, Pennsylvania; June 26, 1972
Tornado—Xenia, Ohio; April 3, 1974
Tornado—Canton, Illinois; July 23, 1975
Subway collision—Boston, Massachusetts; August 1, 1975
Bus crash—Tiffin, Ohio; August 15, 1975
Explosion—Niagara Falls, New York; December 14, 1975
Explosion—Queens, New York; December 29, 1975
Multiple car pile-up—Syracuse, New York; January 2, 1976
Train crash—Chicago, Illinois; January 9, 1976
Explosion, fire—Fremont, Nebraska; January 10, 1976
Nursing home fire—Chicago, Illinois; January 30, 1976
Tornado—Cabot, Arkansas; March 29, 1976
Tornado—Canton, Mississippi; March 30, 1976
Plane crash—St. Thomas, U.S. Virgin Islands; April 27, 1976
Ammonia tanker explosion—Houston, Texas; May 11, 1976
Flood—Teton Dam, Idaho; June 5, 1976
Tornado—Lemont, Illinois; June 13, 1976
Plane crash—Philadelphia, Pennsylvania; June 23, 1976
Explosion—Queens, New York; November 21, 1976
Chlorine threat—Baton Rouge, Louisiana; December 10, 1976
Train wreck—Birmingham, Alabama; January 16, 1976
Explosion—Opelika, Alabama; January 28, 1977
Train crash—Chicago, Illinois; February 4, 1977
Tornadoes—Birmingham, Alabama; April 4, 1977
Plane crash—Atlanta, Georgia; April 5, 1977
Floods—Southeastern West Virginia; April 7, 1977
Floods—Eastern Kentucky; April 8, 1977
Floods—Western Virginia; April 9, 1977
Night club fire—Southgate, Kentucky; May, 1977

Through no fault of the researchers or those from whom they gathered their data, information on the adequacy of triage is sparse and unreliable. Accurate record keeping (with precise times and patient-tracking in the field and in the Emergency Department) is simply not possible in the midst of a mass casualty disaster. Therefore, there is no information on the order in which patients were processed in relation to their diagnosis and prognosis. Although the patients' records do reveal the subsequent hospital diagnoses, no machinery exists to evaluate how reasonable the initial field suppositions were within the limits of time, diagnostic ability, skill levels, and field conditions. In evaluating prehospital care, the question of what the EMT *should* have assumed and done is often more significant than the ultimate definitive diagnosis. For example, the correct field response to tenderness and swelling in a limb is to assume a fracture and to splint. This remains the correct treatment regardless of whether the final hospital diagnosis is a fracture or a bone bruise. In other areas, however, the conclusions of the report are reliable and thorough.

Summarizing a major study in one or 2 pages always involves the risk of oversimplification. However, the following statements drawn from this study are so illustrative as to leave little doubt about its conclusions regarding planning, response, and the quality of patient care:

- "Few community health care systems have undertaken realistic overall planning for handling large numbers of casualties. In over half the communities studied it is generally assumed that everyday EMS can be extended in mass emergencies, i.e., that a system which functions adequately during normal time will also do so in disasters. But our research found that everyday and disaster EMS are *not* simply two points on the same continuum. Mass emergencies create demands that differ qualitatively, as well as quantitatively, from everyday EMS demands."
- ". . . our research suggests that disaster related EMS planning and response is . . . one of the less satisfactory aspects in the provision of EMS in general. The area is marked by lack of knowledge both of disasters and of EMS system operations, by inadequate and incorrect planning, and, especially, by poor response at times of mass emergencies. Response is characterized by inefficiency and ineffectiveness both in processes and in outcomes. . . ."
- "Much of the planning is either inadequate or based on incorrect notions."
- "Response at times of mass emergencies is characterized by lack of overall control and poor communication, resulting in maldistribution of victims and inefficient use of EMS personnel and facilities and with resultant gaps, overlaps, conflicts, etc., among the EMS components involved so as to make suspect the quality of the EMS health care provided."
- "In only about half of the instances studied did the transportation response occur according to any predesignated formal plan. . . ."
- ". . . transporters converged on the scene often in an unsystematic and uncoordinated fashion. This frequently resulted in . . . the less seriously injured patients being transported before those who were more seriously injured."
- "There was a greater tendency to transport victims to hospital facilities immediately rather than to triage and stabilize them at the disaster site. Actual on-site triage occurred in relatively few of the cases examined, with only half of these being done according to some predesignated plan. Even then it was extremely rare that medically trained personnel [EMS personnel of any level/*Ed.*] exercised authority over on-site triage. . . ."

- ". . . in only about one-third of the cases was patient distribution to hospitals done according to some overall plan. . . ."
- ". . . in the majority of these instances over half of the casualties ended up clustered in one hospital."
- "In the events studied, hospitals often failed to receive word of a disaster until the first victims arrived in the ER."
- "In about half of the cases studied there was no evidence of any control or communication structure functioning to organize and coordinate the overall disaster EMS response."
- "In one-half of the events examined, no authority was exercised at all at the disaster site, and in only about one-third of the events was there any overall coordination of the distribution of casualties."
- "The use of communication to achieve coordination was equally rare."
- "Unless pre-impact disagreements over jurisdictions have been settled by prior planning, they may result in absence of coordination, confusion in EMS delivery, and less than satisfactory patient care."
- "In large-scale disasters, the medical problems of casualties tend to involve different degrees of urgency, so the *speed* of the response may not be crucial to effective operations; instead, the overall *coordination* of the response . . . becomes the essential task."
- ". . . we can say that, overall, the delivery of EMS in mass emergencies is not very good, either in absolute or relative terms." [i.e., relative to daily EMS quality/*Ed.*]

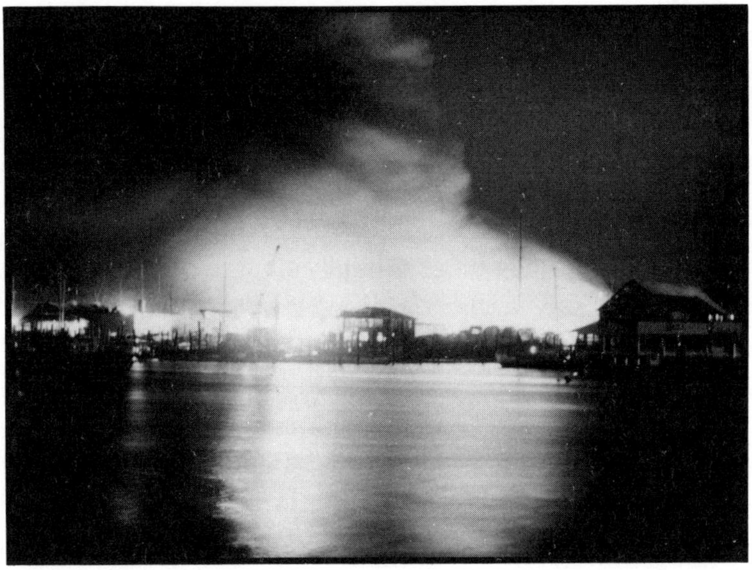

CONCLUSIONS

Neither the polite, dispassionate language of a formal study, nor the often-included scholarly qualifiers, lessen the impact of these evaluations. Simply stated, the Ohio State University study shows that:

1. Most mass casualty planning, response, and patient care is poor—usually well below the daily standards of emergency care.
2. Generally, this is as true in communities *with* plans as in those *without.*
3. This appears to be as true in communities with advanced daily EMS delivery as it is in communities with relatively basic capacities.

We have analyzed many Mass Casualty Incidents since the publication of the Ohio State University study. This was done primarily through a study of accounts in newspapers, often supplemented by lengthy, detailed articles that appeared in the journals, and by papers read at conferences. As one might suspect, the overall conclusion to be drawn is that most areas simply are not prepared to deliver adequate emergency medical care when a Mass Casualty Incident occurs. Furthermore, commonly accepted systems of planning and preparedness seem to be so inappropriate that response is equally poor whether or not there is a plan in place.

It would be an injustice to a group of exceptionally skilled responders not to mention one fact. There *are* instances when the handling of a Mass Casualty Incident has saved countless lives, and where the application of resources, the intervention, the organization, and the field command initiative were of such a high caliber that the response can best be described as a virtuoso performance. When we looked for common denominators in these incidents, we found that there were 2 separate categories. In each category, different factors caused the exceptional response.

Leadership. The incidents in the first category were representative of the usual situations: a plan was in effect with extremely good call-up procedures that assured clear public access and rapid notification of key personnel. Analysis of the plans, however, revealed them to be essentially similar to those that commonly produced unacceptable responses. What then was different? The answer was always clear: *leadership.*

In each of the exemplary responses, either an individual or a group of individuals had shown impressive leadership qualities. The quality of care had been caused, not by the plan but by the field initiative, understanding, and personal leadership skills of these individuals. Generally, they had a predesignated position of authority. However, in one instance, they were simply responders from neighboring areas who filled a leadership function when no predesignated authority arrived or took charge in the field.

It is important to note that these individuals not only had the necessary leadership skills; they also had an understanding of the special needs presented by a mass casualty situation. Furthermore, they were dynamic and effective enough to prevail in the face of difficulties and pressures placed on them by a variety of other factors and authorities.

Urban Response System. The second category of exceptional responses was in urban or highly populated suburban areas. In both locations the magnitude of rapidly available EMS resources, and the structure, response, and command used daily were enough to be effective in a Mass Casualty Incident. These were the underlying causes of the successful response. In these instances field command had definite rank and seemed to be challenged far less than in the non-urban situation.

It is probable that a Mass Casualty Incident in such an urban location must either involve extraordinary conditions or be several times the normal magnitude (200 to 300 victims) before the problems are analogous to those presented in smaller towns by even 25 or 30 victims.

What Does All This Mean?

Any modern EMS system must assume the responsibility of providing adequate emergency care to every patient even at times when there are many patients. It is the patient's *right* to expect essentially the same care in a Mass Casualty Incident as that commonly associated with his or her condition and injuries. What this means is that the system must provide for each patient's stabilization needs regardless of the number of injured. The system, on a patient-by-patient basis, must offer each individual *almost* the same chance of survival he would have if he were the *only* victim. It is clear, however, that most plans do not provide this level of care.

Since it is impractical to expand EMS resources quantitatively, the needs must be met by changing certain factors involved in the response. Most mass casualty plans are made by emergency physicians, nurses, paramedics, and other EMS personnel, including EMTs—all of whom have had sound experience in the daily delivery of emergency care. There is no doubt that their daily activities and interaction with other medical and public safety executives and personnel make them the only group that could create and implement a proper plan.

However, most knowledgeable observers agree that the failure in MCI response generally does not result from inadequacies in fire, rescue, or police functions, but from what is or is not provided for by EMS plans and personnel. Furthermore, it was found that the actual performance of the EMS personnel involved in both adequate and inadequate responses was universally outstanding. Therefore, it becomes apparent that the changes necessary are related neither to police, fire, and rescue operations, nor to the *nature* and *quality* of the EMS responders. Instead, after many years of observation and 3 years of intense analysis and study, we have concluded that the following factors are the causes of generally poor emergency care for the victims of an MCI.

1. **Planners' lack of experience in Mass Casualty Incidents.** The EMS personnel responsible for mass casualty planning lack direct, personal experience of the unique problems involved. Having no secondary sources to use as a guide, they are left with no alternative but to extrapolate their experience and knowledge of daily emergency care into a mass casualty plan. However, experience at Mass Casualty Incidents clearly indicates that the problems are not only *greater* but of a *different nature,* and that mass casualty plans must be *qualitatively* different from plans for daily emergency care. This seems to explain the ineffectiveness of many plans. No group, however clever, can design a strategy for a situation whose elements are unknown to them.

2. **Lack of comparative studies based upon experience.** Available MCI information has not been compiled in a useable, generalized form. Numerous accounts of individual incidents appear in the journals and are presented as papers and lectures at EMS meetings. Although each of these is full of illuminating details, the Ohio State University study is the only work that compares the information from many incidents and generalizes the experience. Further, no work has translated the *collective* experiences into a "response plan"—namely, a general method which can then be adjusted by command personnel to meet each incident's special requirements. Such a general plan would constitute a meaningful matrix, both for the response method and for the responders to understand the events.

3. **Lack of a clear EMS command structure.** A clear EMS command structure is necessary in the field. This does not imply a need for the command to give minute instructions at every step of the way. It simply means that there should be a leader or leaders who can react to special problems and changes in the situation as they arise, and provide guidance to enable EMTs to continue to exercise their own initiative.

4. **Responders' lack of understanding of the unique problems of MCIs.** In most communities, only a few members of the hospital staff and key EMS personnel really understand the overall medical and patient-care ramifications of the mass casualty plan. Certain other individuals with special responsibilities (dispatchers,

directors of Civil Preparedness, etc.), have knowledge of their own immediate area in a Mass Casualty Incident. However, the mass of EMS responders are given no understanding of the goals of a mass casualty plan—they are simply expected to follow orders given to them by those who are in charge.

Thus, the quality of care is adversely affected by the constant need for personnel to be told what to do, and by individuals' inability to exercise their own initiative to achieve common goals. Minimal training devised to provide minimal knowledge without real understanding assures a robot-like and frequently inappropriate response. Any oversight or momentary confusion on the part of the leaders under this system, is apt to result in haul-and-run chaos.

All EMS personnel must have an overall view and understanding of the special situations they will encounter in a Mass Casualty Incident, and of the special techniques that are required to deal with these situations.

This text has been written to provide a basis for the resolution of these problems.

Chapter 2
DEFINING A "MASS CASUALTY INCIDENT"

What Is an MCI?

The initiating mechanisms of disasters that produce large numbers of victims can vary greatly: floods, earthquakes, fires, explosions, plane crashes, and so on. It is therefore important to define *Mass Casualty Incident* within the context of this book.

The common differentiation between *man-made* disasters and *acts of nature* is not pertinent for a discussion of the resulting EMS problems. Neither is a categorization based upon number of patients. However, whether the problem is unique and localized, or whether it affects a broad geographical area is highly pertinent. For example, a flood involving several counties presents different EMS problems than does a train crash. While it is true that floods, blizzards, and similar environmental disasters increase emergency medical needs, cause local resources to be stressed, and require alteration of normal EMS systems, these types of disasters generally do not produce a large number of patients *all needing stabilization at one time and in one place.* This book does not deal with these geographically widespread disasters. It is limited to what we have designated *Mass Casualty Incidents* (MCIs).

MCIs are disasters that occur in one location in the absence of similar or related occurrences in neighboring towns or counties. The incidents we are considering have a common location and time of insult for all involved patients.

In order to plan an effective response that will provide for EMS needs, one must first determine what these needs are likely to be. One must, upon a broad base of experience, determine:

What is likely to occur?
When?
Where?
Of what magnitude?
Of what medical nature?

Twenty-two Case Histories

Over the last 3 years a staff team has compiled and studied information on 22 nonenvironmental disasters (MCIs). Each staff member has had professional experience in this type of research in EMS, in education, and in training. While some of our work was statistical, most of it dealt with getting an in-depth understanding of what happened. We read accounts of each MCI, attended presentations on the incidents, and questioned those who analyzed the responses. We were always guided by the questions raised and by what we knew or had already studied. The most significant aspect of the work was that we were *comparing* MCIs.

As general patterns emerged, and we re-examined each incident to see if the patterns held up, we found that certain interesting observations could be based on this varied group of MCIs. Bear in mind, however, that our sample was not scientifically selected. The incidents included were those that received coverage in the national press and at major disaster conferences. Since small MCIs (15 to 25 victims) rarely receive such coverage, our study is heavily weighted toward larger incidents.

Weather and season. The MCIs in our study took place in a wide variety of weather conditions, and were scattered throughout the seasons of the year. Few of the 22 incidents occurred during what might be considered adverse conditions.

Light/dark and time of day. Although incidents seemed to cluster slightly, they occurred throughout the 24 hours of the day.

Ignition. Six incidents owed their start to fire.

Population density. Any attempt to group the incidents by population density proved meaningless. For example, a bus accident may have taken place in a rural setting far from the city center, but *within* the city limits. Therefore, it is misleading to say that the accident happened in a city of 150,000 people. Furthermore, incidents may not actually take place in the town or city to which they are attributed. Plane crashes, in particular, are often listed as occurring in the city of destination. (The "Portland" plane crash actually happened in a town some distance from Portland. Therefore, to say that the accident happened in a city of 380,000 is thoroughly misleading.)

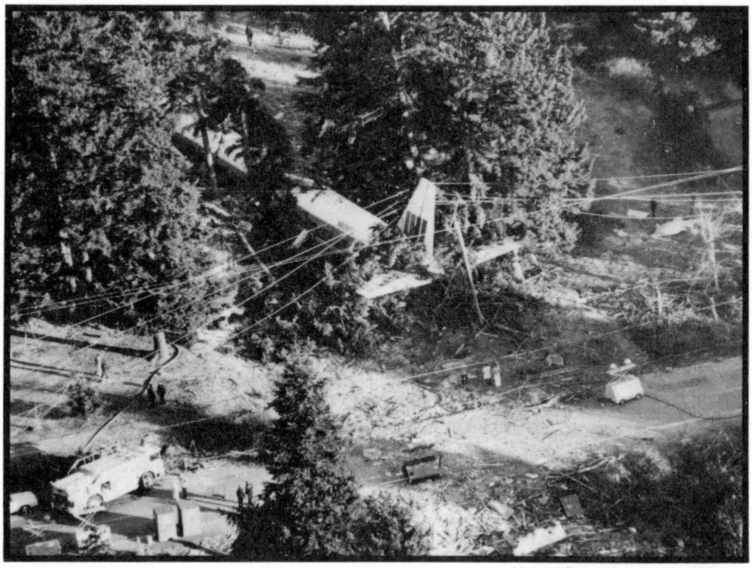

United Press International Photo

What can be said about population in relation to MCIs is that some of the incidents in our sample occurred in larger metropolitan areas, some in small cities, some in towns, and some in rural areas.

Type of incident. There were 12 incidents related to transportation, 9 of which involved transport of people. Of the 9, 4 were commuter-related.

Nine incidents were related to buildings where large groups of people were gathered. Three incidents were related to hazardous materials. (Two of of these were also related to transportation.)

Victims. Eight incidents had more than 80 victims; 9 incidents involved 40 to 80 victims; and 5 incidents had fewer than 40. It may be noted that no matter how many victims were involved overall, most of the *major* incidents studied produced 40 to 80 patients with serious multiple injuries and systemic complications. In incidents involving greater numbers of people, it was found that there were higher numbers of dead, and/or there were higher numbers of low-priority patients whose injuries were localized. In no case did the number of seriously injured survivors rise above 120.

OBSERVATIONS

Our observations, based upon 22 MCIs and the Ohio State University study, are as follows:

1. An MCI can happen at any time of the day or night, at any season of the year, in any part of the country, and in communities both large and small.
2. If an area transports children to school in buses; if there is a highway or railroad tracks running through a town; if there are commuters to or from a town; if a town is on the banks of a river; if it is located under or near a flight path (and there is practically no place in America that isn't)—then there is a chance of a major transportation-related disaster.
3. If a town has buildings where large groups of people gather—hotels, schools, churches, shopping centers, apartment buildings, auditoriums, etc.—then there is a chance of a building-related MCI.
4. If any businesses in an area make, use, or store hazardous materials (grain elevators, factories, warehouses, etc.) or if hazardous materials are ever transported near or through a town, then there is a chance of a hazardous-materials-related disaster.
5. If an MCI does occur, there is the highest probability of having from 40 to 80 seriously injured people to treat. To preplan for any lesser number is to invite failure.

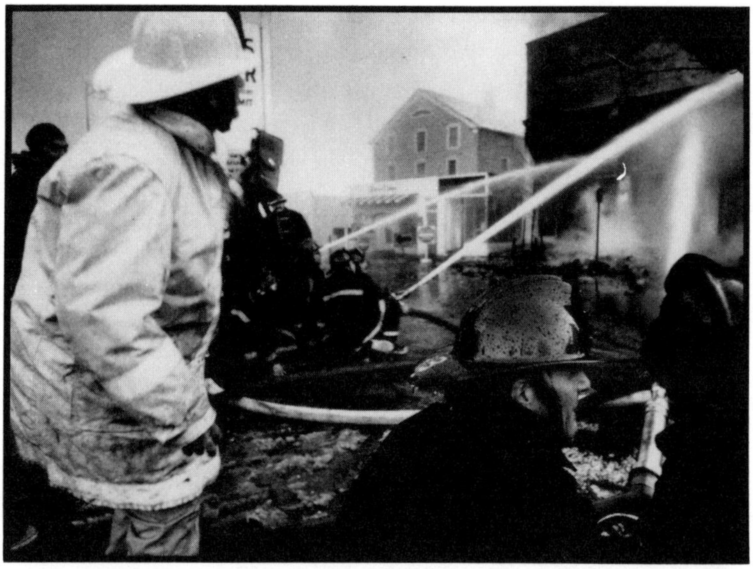

We feel that these observations apply equally to small farming communities and major metropolises. It is foolish to suppose, for any reason, that a Mass Casualty Incident "can't happen here." It *can*! The only questions are, "*When* will it happen?" and "Will you be prepared?" Every community should have a response plan and properly trained personnel ready to go into action when an MCI becomes a reality.

The following table is a summary of the data surrounding the 22 incidents. The reader will find studying it—and the synopsis of each of the 22 incidents that follows—a worthwhile familiarization exercise before going further in the text.

INCIDENT	LOCATION	DATE
1. Train crash	Chicago, IL	Oct. 30, '72
2. High-rise collapse	Fairfax, VA	Mar. 2, '73
3. Bomb explosion, airport	Queens, NY	Dec. 29, '75
4. Supper club fire	Southgate, KY	May 25, '77
5. County jail fire	Columbia, TN	June 26, '77
6. Prison fire	Danbury, CT	July 7, '77
7. Grain elevator explosion	Westwego, LA	Dec. 22, '77
8. Propane tanker explosion	Waverly, TN	Feb. 24, '78
9. Truck explosion	New York, NY	June 20, '78
10. Ferryboat crash	New York, NY	Nov. 28, '78
11. Airliner crash	Portland, OR	Dec. 28, '78
12. Elevated train crash	Chicago, IL	Feb. 4, '77
13. Airliner crash	Chicago, IL	May 25, '79
14. Bus collision,	Rye,NY	July, 3, '79
15. Bus collision	Bethesda, MD	July 21, '79
16. Stampede at rock concert	Cincinnati, OH	Dec. 3, '79
17. Ship-bridge collision	Tampa Bay, FL	May 9, '80
18. Hotel fire	Las Vegas, NV	Nov. 21 '80
19. Hotel fire	Harrison, NY	Dec. 3, '80
20. Train crash	Staten Island, NY	Dec. 29, '80
21. Subway train crash	New York, NY	July 3, '81
22. Building collapse	Kansas City, MO	July 17, '81

TIME	WEATHER	VICTIMS	INJURED	DEAD
7:35 AM	n/f	364	320	44
2:20 PM	n/f	78	64	14
6:33 PM	n/f	86	75	11
8:45 PM	clear (n/f)	235 +	70 +	167
1:55 PM	n/f	75	33	42
1:30 AM	n/f	71	66	5
9:10 AM	n/f	49	13	36
2:59 PM	mild (n/f)	115	90	25
1:30 PM	clear (n/f)	106	106	0
8:00 AM	fog	160	160	0
6:14 PM	cold (n/f)	70	60	10
5:30 PM	snow	172	160	12
3:04 PM	rain (n/f)	273	0	273
Afternoon	n/f	45	45	0
5:30 AM	n/f	38	38	0
7:00 PM	n/f	19	8	11
7:33 PM	fog, rain, wind	33	1	32
7:10 AM	clear (n/f)	784	700	84
10:20 AM	cold (n/f)	56	30	26
8:03 AM	fog	80	80	0
1:50 PM	n/f	135–150	134–149	1
7:01 PM	n/f	299 +	188 +	111

n/f: not a factor

Train Crash **Chicago, IL** **7:30 AM, October 30, 1972**

A double-decker train was backing up after having overshot its station during the morning rush hour, when another train crashed into its rear car. The 2 colliding cars virtually collapsed on contact. Many people were trapped in the wreckage and it took several hours to extricate them all. The crash occurred only 200 yards from one hospital and a few blocks from another. Hospital doctors and nurses responded directly to the scene.

Time of year: fall
Time of day: morning—daylight
Weather: not a factor
Victims: 364
Dead: 44
Injured: 320

High-Rise Collapse **Fairfax, VA** **2:20 PM, March 2, 1973**

Concrete had recently been poured on the twenty-fifth floor of a high-rise building under construction. When this floor buckled and fell, a major portion of the building came crashing down—floor after floor. A 3-level parking lot attached to the building also collapsed. As the collapse began, workmen were alerted and started running from the building. Some jumped from high floors, but many could not get out.

Time of year: winter
Time of day: afternoon—daylight
Weather: not a factor
Victims: 78
Dead: 14
Injured: 64

Bomb Explosion Queens, NY 6:33 PM, December 29, 1975

A bomb estimated to have the power of 25 sticks of dynamite exploded in a locker at a crowded baggage claim area at La Guardia Airport. The ceiling of the area collapsed and shattered glass flew in all directions. The baggage area was especially crowded due to holiday travelers.

Time of year: winter
Time of day: evening—darkness
Weather: not a factor
Victims: 86
Dead: 11
Injured: 75

Supper Club Fire Southgate, KY 8:45 PM, May 25, 1977

The Beverly Hills Supper Club was a major entertainment center. Basically a one-floor building, it covered approximately 1-½ acres and contained several different rooms for dining and entertainment. The largest of the rooms held 1,200 to 1,300 people at the time the fire began, shortly before the evening show. The cause is believed to have been electrical. It started in a concealed area and had time to develop before being observed. All of the deaths that occurred were attributed to smoke inhalation. The number of people in the club was about double the number the building could safely accommodate. The number in the main room where most deaths occurred was about triple the safe level.

Time of year: spring
Time of day: evening—dusk
Weather: not a factor
Victims: 235 +
Dead: 167
Injured: 70 known, assumed higher

County Jail Fire **Columbia, TN** **1:55 PM, June 26, 1977**

The fire was deliberately set by an inmate in a padded cell about 20 feet down the hall from the visiting room, which contained 40 to 50 visitors and about 30 prisoners. The cell padding was the only thing that burned in the one-story fireproof building. The county medical examiner suggested that there may have been a toxic agent in the smoke that was the primary cause of the deaths, rather than simple smoke inhalation. There was great difficulty in evacuating the prisoners because when the visitors rushed the exits, the keys to the cellblock were lost for about 12 minutes. The dead included 34 prisoners and 8 visitors.

Time of year: summer
Time of day: afternoon—daylight
Weather: not a factor
Victims: 75
Dead: 42
Injured: 33

Prison Fire **Danbury, CT** **1:30 AM, July 7, 1977**

A flash fire moved quickly through the second floor of a 3-story cellblock at the Federal Correctional Institution. Firemen had some trouble entering the area because of locked gates. Many inmates were trapped on the second floor; some were rescued from there by a hook and ladder. The 5 deaths were attributed to smoke inhalation.

Time of year: summer
Time of day: night—darkness
Weather: not a factor
Victims: 71
Dead: 5
Injured: 66

Grain Elevator Explosion Westwego, LA 9:10 AM, Dec. 22, 1977

A group of 73 silos was hit by a chain reaction of explosions that destroyed 45 of the units. Many of the dead and injured were in a two-story office building on the site that was crushed by the huge quantities of falling concrete and steel. Others were trapped on top of burning platforms. The grain dust explosion was believed to have started in the weighing station, possibly ignited by a spark from a conveyor belt.

Time of year: winter
Time of day: morning—daylight
Weather: not a factor
Victims: 49
Dead: 36*
Injured: 13

*Most of the dead were found in the slow process of removing debris.

Propane Tanker Explosion Waverly, TN 2:59 PM, Feb. 24, 1978

Twenty-four cars of a 92-car train derailed in a mixed commercial/residential section of a small town. Two of the cars were liquid propane tankers. There was no explosion, fire, or spill at the time of the derailment. During the next 40 hours clean-up operations went ahead. Many residents were evacuated from the area, though some had returned. Suddenly, one of the tankers ruptured and ignited, creating a huge fireball which "leveled" a 3-block area. Many police, fire, safety, and railroad officials were at the site when the explosion occurred and were among the dead (including the police and fire chiefs) and the badly injured. Most victims suffered from burns, possibly being first sprayed with liquid propane and then ignited. Fire continued for several hours after the explosion. The tankers had been continuously checked for leaks by experts from the time of derailment to the time of the explosion.

Time of year: winter
Time of day: afternoon—daylight
Weather: clear/mild (not a factor)
Victims: 115
Dead: 25
Injured: 90

Truck Explosion New York, NY 1:30 PM, June 20, 1978

An ice cream truck exploded at a busy intersection in the Wall Street area of New York City. The truck was carrying a 2-½ gallon can of gasoline with a rag stuffed in the opening. The driver saw a fire begin and stopped the truck. The gas can then exploded, and shortly after, the truck's gas tank. The explosion sent debris flying and blew out windows on many surrounding buildings. Most injuries were from flying glass.

Time of year: summer
Time of day: afternoon—daylight
Weather: clear (not a factor)
Victims: 106
Dead: 0
Injured: 106

Ferryboat Crash New York, NY 8:00 AM, November 8, 1978

A ferry from Staten Island was carrying about 2,000 passengers to Manhattan in a dense fog. Visibility was near zero and radar was being used. The boat missed its docking area by 700 feet and crashed into a wall at about 5 knots. Most of the injured were walking on the decks when the accident occurred. It was about 15 minutes before the boat was able to tie up at the dock.

Time of year: autumn
Time of day: morning—daylight
Weather: fog (significant factor)
Victims: 160
Dead: 0
Injured: 160

Airliner Crash Portland, OR 6:14 PM, December 28, 1978

A DC-8 ran out of fuel while circling near the Portland airport because of a failure to confirm that its landing gear was down. The pilot attempted to put down in a dark area amid the many lights of a "crowded residential area" on the edge of the city. The plane landed on 2 houses in which no one was home. It narrowly missed an apartment building with about 500 tenants. No one on the ground was injured. There was no ignition upon crash. Passengers had been prepared for a no-gear landing. Only the fire department had been notified by the airport of a possible crash landing.

Time of year: winter
Time of day: evening—darkness
Weather: not a factor
Victims: 70
Dead: 10
Injured: 60

Elevated Train Crash Chicago, IL 5:30 PM, February 4, 1977

The elevated train was crowded with rush-hour passengers when it came around a curve and ran into the back of another train. Two cars fell 20 feet to the street, landing on their sides. The rear end of another fell to the street while its front end remained on the track. A fourth car did not fall but struck a girder and was held partway on the track.

Time of year: winter
Time of day: afternoon—dusk
Weather: snow
Victims: 172
Dead: 12
Injured: 160

Airliner Crash **Chicago, IL** **3:04 PM, May 25, 1979**

As Flight 191 for Los Angeles traveled down the runway for takeoff, its left engine separated from the aircraft and was left on the ground. The plane lifted off, banked sharply, and crashed to the ground at a near-vertical angle. It came down in a field only a few yards from a mobile home park. The crash and explosion were so severe that there were no survivors. No one on the ground was injured. The location of the crash was very fortunate considering the many factories and offices nearby.

Time of year: spring
Time of day: afternoon—daylight
Weather: not a factor
Victims: 273
Dead: 273
Injured: 0

Bus Collision **Rye, NY** **Afternoon, July 3, 1979**

Two buses were traveling together, taking children from a Head Start program to an amusement park. When the lead bus stopped for a light, the second bus ran into it. (The driver said that the brakes had failed.) All injuries were on the second bus, including 3 brothers described as hemophiliacs.

Time of year: summer
Time of day: afternoon—daylight
Weather: not a factor
Victims: 45
Dead: 0
Injured: 45

Bus Collision Bethesda, MD 5:30 AM, July 21, 1979

A bus without passengers skidded around a corner, crossed the center line, and hit an oncoming bus head on. The second bus was carrying 40 passengers, almost all of whom had some injury. Most were treated for cuts, bruises, and fractures.

Time of year: summer
Time of day: morning—daylight
Weather: not a factor
Victims: 38
Dead: 0
Injured: 38

Stampede at Rock Concert Cincinnati, OH 7:00 PM, Dec. 3, 1979

Most of the 18,348 tickets for the concert were for first-come-first-served seating. People began lining up outside hours before the 8:00 PM starting time. Though the doors are usually opened at 6:00 PM for the concerts in this arena, that night they did not open until just after 7:00. About 10 percent of the audience was lined up at the doors where the accident occurred. Sounds of music apparently led some to believe that the concert had begun. When the doors were opened, the crowd stampeded in. Many fell and could not get up. All the fatalities were caused by asphyxiation.

Time of year: fall
Time of day: evening—dark
Weather: not a factor
Victims: 19
Dead: 11
Injured: 8

Ship-Bridge Collision **Tampa Bay, FL** **7:33 AM, May 9, 1980**

The Sunshine Skyway is a 15-mile chain of 5 bridges and 6 causeways stretching across Tampa Bay. In a thick fog, with thunder showers and high winds, a 609-foot freighter crashed into a bridge abutment. A 1300-foot stretch of roadway collapsed and fell 140 feet into the water. A Greyhound bus with 23 aboard, 3 cars, and a pickup truck also fell. Only the driver of the truck survived. The bus sank in 20 feet of water on top of the cars.

Time of year: spring
Time of day: morning—daylight
Weather: fog, rain, high winds (causative factor)
Victims: 33
Dead: 32
Injured: 1

Hotel Fire **Las Vegas, NV** **7:10 AM, November 21, 1980**

The fire began in the ceiling of the ground floor, most of which was occupied by the casino and a restaurant. Because it was early morning there were relatively few people present. The fire spread "within a few minutes" across the entire ground floor. The resulting smoke traveled up elevator shafts and stairwells to the 26 floors above. It was estimated that 7,000 to 8,000 people were in the hotel at the time. Two hundred were picked off the roof by helicopter.

Time of year: fall
Time of day: morning—daylight
Weather: clear (not a factor)
Victims: 784
Dead: 84
Injured: 700

Hotel Fire **Harrison, NY** **10:20 AM, December 3, 1980**

The Stouffer's Inn was crowded with executives from several corporations, gathered for business meetings. Suddenly, on one corner of the building's third floor, thick, blinding smoke appeared, and within seconds fire flashed through a 100-foot section of the building. Fire regulations did not require sprinklers in that area of the hotel. Some survivors leaped 35 feet to a rocky slope, suffering injuries in the process. Some bodies were found in a closet that had been mistaken for an exit; others were found by a bolted exit. The cause was determined to be arson.

Time of year: winter
Time of day: morning
Weather: not a factor
Victims: 56
Dead: 26
Injured: 30

Train Crash **Staten Island, NY** **8:03 AM, December 29, 1980**

A 4-car train failed to stop at its station and continued into a brick wall during rush hour. Though the tracks were reported to be wet due to recent heavy fog, it was undetermined whether the brakes had been applied or not. Many of the passengers were standing at the time of the crash, as they prepared to get off the train.

Time of year: winter
Time of day: morning—daylight
Weather: fog
Victims: 80
Dead: 0
Injured: 80

Subway Train Crash New York, NY 1:50 PM, July 3, 1981

A 10-car subway, travelling at about 15 miles per hour, slammed into the rear of another 10-car train that had halted for signal trouble in a darkened tunnel in Brooklyn. The impact hurled passengers to the floor, and left the front of the following train crumpled up to the first door. The motorman of the following train died of his injuries shortly before he was extricated at 6:00 PM. Between 135 and 150 patients were treated by rescue workers at 4 nearby hospitals.

Time of year: summer
Time of day: afternoon—daytime; but underground, in darkness
Weather: not a factor
Victims: 135–150
Dead: 1
Injured: 134–149

Building Collapse Kansas City, MO 7:01 PM, July 17, 1981

Fifteen hundred people were dancing at the nearly-new Hyatt-Regency Hotel. Up to 150 were dancing on 2 concrete walkways suspended over the dance floor. Suddenly a walkway collapsed, fell onto the second walkway directly below, and both went crashing to the ground floor. Broken gas pipes threatened explosions, hampering initial rescue efforts. Heavy machinery was required to remove debris from victims trapped under and between the walkways. Rescue efforts could not be completed until 12 hours had passed.

Time of year: summer
Time of day: evening
Weather: not a factor
Victims: 299 +
Dead: 111
Injured: 188 +

Chapter 3

UNIVERSAL PROBLEMS AND RESPONSE FAILURES

Patterns of Response

One might suppose that Mass Casualty Incidents are so diverse and bizarre that they are unpredictable. The Ohio State University study clearly indicates that when generalizations are based upon *daily* EMS, this supposition is correct. However, study of field experience with MCIs reveals the following:

1. The events are predictable.
2. The chain of events is predictable.
3. The problems are predictable.
4. The failures are predictable.

This is true because regardless of the initiating mechanisms, human behavior and the basic EMS needs are predictable. Anyone involved in combat or any other form of crisis activity knows that a group's response to stress is uncannily consistent. The cast of characters and the development of the drama are repeated with the consistency of a "sociological law"; the only unpredictable variant is, which individual will assume which role.

A hypothetical chain of events can serve to illustrate this point. Assume that you are a reporter, untrained in assisting, and can only observe and record. A school bus carrying 48 children is in an accident. It rolls down an embankment. Rapidly, word gets out that 4 children are dead, 12 to 18 are critically injured, and that only 3 or 4 children are unhurt. You observe the responders, the problems, the parents, the bystanders. When the field is cleared you go to the near hospitals, interview people, and watch the reactions and dramas that unfold. Later you compile all your notes into an article. Subsequently, you witness the same incident in 9 other communities located throughout the country. None of the communities are alike. Some are rural, some suburban, some urban. Some are wealthy, some poor. They represent different regional and geophysical environments. Each time you observe, record, and write an article.

What differences in problems, human behavior, and human reactions do you think you would find? The answer is *very little*.

Similarly, by observing drills we have found common responder-performance patterns. In a school bus MCI simulation, for example, if not told where to go, or if not regulated, everyone tries to get on the bus. At drills where no command is established (or where it has been purposely withdrawn at the time when 5 or 6 crews arrive), the result is always the same. The crews stand around for a few seconds undecided. Then they disperse in groups to the nearest and most critically hurt victims. They stabilize and treat these, load them 2 to 3 in each ambulance, and head for the nearest hospital, carrying all of their equipment with them.

This behavior is repeated at any drill where neither command nor adequate training of personnel has occurred. Unfortunately, this also occurs at many Mass Casualty Incidents.

Once one realizes the predictability of human reactions and the specific patient-care needs, one can establish a plan. This plan will produce the behavior modification necessary to meet the patients' needs and will reduce morbidity and mortality.

Two facts explain why responders to an MCI have been unable to analyze their responses and detail what went wrong. First, few EMS executives find it possible to discuss publicly what went wrong. Second, a serious public study of response failures and preplanning failures could result in lawsuits against the municipality or county involved. The combination of the emotional and legal climate that follows a mass casualty response results in a feeling of camaraderie, fostering the conclusion that "We did a great job, though we had a few minor problems." Such a climate is not conducive to careful critical analysis.

The Ohio State study provided a basis for us. Finally, we were able to synthesize the observed failures. We then analyzed these failures at a wide variety of drills and exercises.

The following problems were displayed over and over again. They were so common that one must assume they will be present at future Mass Casualty Incidents *unless specifically addressed in preplanning and training*.

Problems Found at Most Mass Casualty Incidents

1. Failure in adequate alerting
2. Lack of rapid "primary" stabilization of all patients
3. Failure to rapidly move, collect, and organize patients at a suitable place
4. Failure to provide proper (or any) triage
5. Use of overly time-consuming and inappropriate care methods
6. Premature commencement of transportation
7. Improper use of personnel in the field
8. Lack of proper distribution of patients, resulting in improper use of medical facilities
9. Lack of recognizable EMS command in the field
10. Lack of proper preplanning and lack of adequate training of *all* personnel
11. Failure to compensate for malfunction and remediate problems
12. Lack of adequate or proper communication

1. **Failure in adequate alerting**. In most incidents there was a failure in rapid, sensibly sequenced alerting of all key personnel. Commonly, a random EMS response left vast areas uncovered, causing delay and unnecessarily long initial response times. Seldom were all potentially necessary hospitals alerted early. Also common were hospitals that received no alerting at all and first learned of the situation when patients appeared at the Emergency Department. Call-up plans often were not rigid; instead, there was *ad libbing* by dispatchers. Since they often lacked good citizen access or crossover, the first emergency agency notified usually could not trigger call-up.

2. **Lack of rapid "primary" stabilization of all patients.** Almost no response could be found where a significant primary scan of all patients was completed by the earliest responders to arrive—a lack that could have resulted in loss of life.

3. **Failure to rapidly move, collect, and organize patients at a suitable place**. Very few incidents showed any central collecting station and treatment center at the site. Generally, patients were treated where they lay. In closed situations the space was inappropriate for proper care, and dangerous. In open situations the vastness resulted in random selection based upon location. In both instances, since patients were not moved to a central location, they could not be efficiently retriaged and cared for. Even in cases when a collecting station *was* established (rare as they were), too much care was administered to patients where they lay.

4. **Failure to provide proper (or any) triage**. In most cases, *no* triage occurred at all. When triage did occur, it was performed

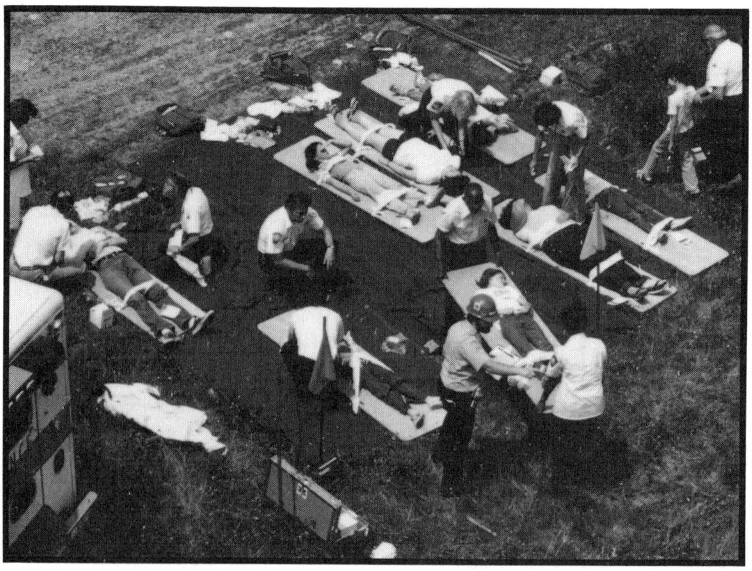

on a daily EMS basis rather than a mass casualty basis. This resulted in diverting care and assets to the catastrophically injured, most of whom died. This means that others who had a good chance, if given care, died needlessly.

5. **Use of overly time-consuming and inappropriate care methods**. Use of daily considerations and methods proved terribly time consuming and usually resulted in poor treatment. Carefully detailed assessment of a multitrauma victim is often misleading in prehospital care. Instead, one must *assume* multiple fractures that cannot adequately be located in the field. Long-boarding in a normal anatomical position is faster and supports the entire body, without excessive localized pressure.

6. **Premature commencement of transportation**. Commonly, the first 4 or 5 ambulances to arrive left before all patients had been stabilized and before enough personnel and equipment were available in the field. Ironically, they usually transported dead and/or moribund patients, and arrived at a near hospital before sufficient time had elapsed to allow upstaffing of the key departments. In short, premature transportation resulted in unnecessary, critical understaffing in the field. It also focused care on a small, generally unsalvageable group while others received none; and it taxed hospitals before they were ready to provide proper care.

7. **Improper use of personnel in the field**. In areas where only BLS was supplied, IV and ALS teams were usually not brought rapidly to the field. Physicians present attempted to administrate instead of assuming ALS treatment assignments. Where mixed ALS and BLS response existed, ALS personnel were frequently not directed to concentrate on ALS skills. Instead, BLS personnel were at the collecting station, while some ALS personnel were doing BLS tasks.

8. **Lack of proper distribution of patients, resulting in improper use of medical facilities**. Too often, most of the patients from an incident were transported to the near hospital regardless of its stabilization capacity, even when other hospitals were only 5 to 10 minutes farther from the site. Because the near hospital couldn't handle the patient load, other victims (regardless of their condition) were transported up to 2 hours from the site without retriage or additional care. Although each community had different geographic situations in regard to near and far hospitals, rarely were patients well distributed either quantitatively or qualitatively.

9. **Lack of recognizable EMS command in the field**. In most cases *no* medical command existed in the field. When it did, the command personnel were almost impossible to locate or identify. In other incidents a variety of EMS executives took charge, resulting in too many commanders and no effective control. Generally, command, if established at all, became recognizable

very late in the incident, after the point when it could contribute to orderly operations and salvage. Lack of command resulted in confusion, contradictory actions, inability to adjust or remediate problems, and a lack of necessary field initiative. Although inappropriate in every case, it was not uncommon to find an attempt at control from another location such as a hospital. Medical command and initiative *must* be at the site.

10. **Lack of proper preplanning and lack of adequate training of all personnel**. In almost no single location were we able to find all responders, physicians, and key hospital personnel well trained in either an overview, or in their own parts of the mass casualty response. The Ohio State study indicates almost no difference in quality of care whether or not plans existed. This is not surprising since most preplanning is unrealistic and done by people without experience. Failure of realistic preplanning and training of *all* personnel results in confusion, inappropriate actions, and the need for unnecessarily strong and structured command (usually not possible) at the disaster site. This also results in terribly inefficient operations, much yelling of orders, and unnecessary confusion and excitement. Lack of preplanning and training also results in the making of more on-the-spot command decisions than are necessary (i.e., inherent in the situation). This burden results in many incorrect and improper decisions.

11. **Failure to compensate for malfunction and remediate problems**. When field triage and distribution failed, the hospital receiving the patient overload usually compounded the error by "going ahead faster," instead of retriaging and redistributing to other medical facilities. Compensating actions to offset malfunction of the response were extremely rare. Nor was there rapid remediation of the problems.

12. **Lack of adequate or proper communication**. Generally, not enough significant communication occured. Hospitals neither received nor gave status reports. Worse, often the communication was pre-emptive, such as, "Don't send any more patients here." The problem was not lack of radios or equipment; it lay in the people communicating—or rather, *not* communicating.

CONCLUSION

Noting the consistent reoccurrence of these problems, one can devise a general plan, including a training program, that will address them effectively. The plan, and specific subjects enlarged on in the ensuing chapters, have been isolated specifically for this purpose.

Chapter 4
DETAILING SPECIAL NEEDS

Daily EMS and MCI Care Compared

In a mass casualty disaster, which instantly produces 15 to 80 or more patients, a special group of needs is presented that is generally outside the training of most EMS personnel. Yet, even in this situation, each patient has the right to expect reliable emergency medical care.

The underlying principle of normal, daily EMS care is to meet the medical needs of the patient from the earliest possible moment after the emergency, until definitive medical treatment can be provided. In practice, this care involves a great number of people. We frequently overpower the problem with personnel. The victim of a motor vehicle accident often has 25 or more fire, rescue, police, and EMS responders working to safeguard, extricate, evaluate, stabilize, package, treat, and transport him. A team of doctors, nurses, and EMTs may be assembled to provide care in the Emergency Department. Operating Room and Intensive Care Unit teams then take over. Laboratory technicians, X-ray technicians, respiratory technicians, and consulting physicians are also involved. In a 2-hour period, as many as 80 to 100 people may focus their attention on a single patient's needs.

At the onset of a Mass Casualty Incident, however, there is a sustained period of time in which patients outnumber responding EMTs by a sizable margin. Not until 20 minutes to an hour later, and then only in the best of situations, is there a likelihood of establishing a ratio of one EMT to one patient.

The sustained period of time in which the ratio of emergency personnel to patients is critically different from the "normal" emergency situation, establishes the need for a special program.

Mutual Aid or Mass Casualty Response?

In order to determine which situations necessitate the use of a *mass casualty response* and which can be handled with a standard *mutual aid response*, it is essential to have a reliable definition of each. A quantitative definition—such as, "Any incident with more than 15 seriously injured patients is an MCI"—is incomplete and does not provide reliable criteria. For example, a given unit, the neighboring ambulance squads, and the local hospital may be able to handle 10 multiple-trauma patients within the scope of normal mutual aid. But if 8 of the 10 have severe thoracic injury, it is unlikely that proper care can be provided.

Other factors are also involved. Weather conditions can have a significant effect on both the speed with which responders reach the disaster site and their ability to administer proper care. The remoteness of the site and the nature of the terrain are also factors. All these things, not simply the number of injured, must be considered in determining the type of response that is needed. The vital indexes in this judgment are *time* and *resources*.

MUTUAL AID RESPONSE

A mutual aid response will be adequate if:

1. First Responders and the responding EMS squad can mitigate life threat to the usually accepted level;
2. *and*, within 10 to 20 minutes, enough other responders and ambulances can be at the site to provide normal levels of care and transportation;
3. *and*, the hospitals that can be reached within the normally accepted patient-transport time can provide adequate patient stabilization until definitive care can be provided.

The use of a mutual aid rather than a mass casualty response also requires preplanning, good alerting and communication, discipline, and the establishment of patient treatment and transportation priorities. It may be necessary for the near hospital to activate *its* disaster plan, even though it was not necessary to invoke a mass casualty response in the field.

A MASS CASUALTY INCIDENT

A Mass Casualty Incident exists when:

1. the number of patients and the nature of their injuries make the normal level of stabilization and care unachievable;
2. *and/or*, the number of EMTs and ambulances that can be brought to the field within the time allowed is not enough;
3. *and/or*, the stabilization capabilities of the hospitals that can be reached within the time allowed are insufficient to handle all the patients.

In a Mass Casualty Incident, the quantity of personnel and resources *ultimately* available is insignificant. Only those available *within the allowable time period* are of value. If this quantity is below the requirements for a normal level of patient stabilization, *qualitative* changes in method and structure must be employed. Enlargement plans are not sufficient if time problems are involved.

Mass Casualty Plans

A mass casualty plan must be simple. Elaborate, highly detailed plans will prove unworkable and will result in confusion when an incident occurs. A plan that spells out excessive detail for each possible contingency is difficult to coordinate. It can neither be efficiently looked up nor be remembered by responding personnel. *If the plan cannot be outlined in 2 or 3 pages*, it is unlikely that responders will be able to remember it. If most responding personnel cannot retain and describe the plan from memory, with some accuracy, *it will not operate efficiently*.

A good plan *does* have a detailed, precise call-up and alerting system. Beyond that, it has a structure for general organization and communication that is clear-cut, but *not* developed in detail. It presents a *general method* that is applicable to *any* mass casualty situation, and relies on the training and knowledge of responding personnel to apply and adjust the method to the specific incident involved. Each mass casualty involves constantly changing needs that are impossible to foresee in detailed preplanning, and that are best handled by on-the-scene command personnel. A good field command will redirect resources as problems arise, using the clearly established communications system.

Who's in Charge?

The most significant aspect of preplanning is the assignment of responsibility and authority. An analysis of problems encountered in actual incident responses and drills shows that the problems themselves, and/or the inability to surmount them, were primarily due to a lack of clarity in the assignment of authority, a failure to recognize the *need* for assigning certain authority, or clearly inappropriate assignment of authority.

The question of who has *overall* authority and responsibility is a simple one because it is answered in basically the same manner in each state's statutes. The chief executive of the town, city, or county has both the responsibility and full authority. The chief executive has daily interaction with the public safety officers. Since he or she is accustomed to delegating authority and is rarely trained in line command of fire, police, rescue, or EMS matters, there is usually a clear division of responsibility and a minimum of conflicting orders. The local chief executive remains in charge unless the governor formally declares a state of emergency, in which case the governor and the appropriate state agencies assume the responsibility and take command.

The question of line command responsibility for each major group of responders is usually clear-cut. The fire chief is in charge of fire prevention and suppression, and of all fire personnel. The police chief is in charge of crowd control, traffic, civil order, and all police personnel. Depending on the state statutes, either the police chief or the fire chief is charged with public safety at the site. He

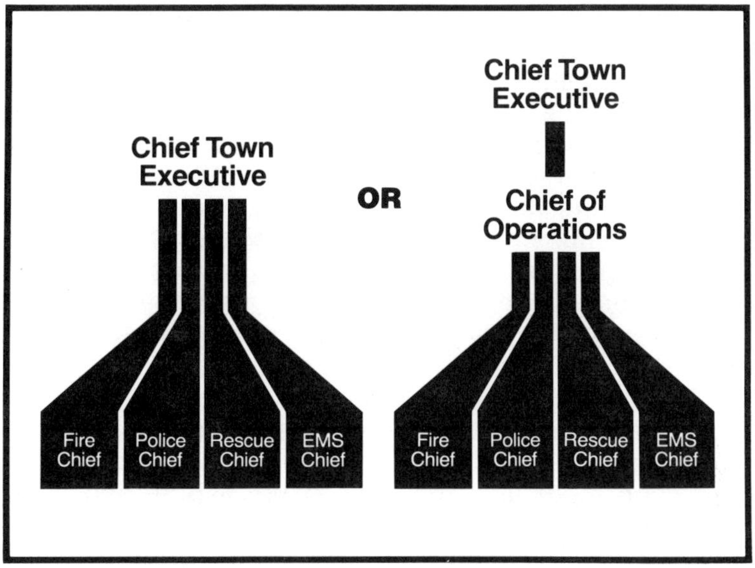

must determine whether it is safe to proceed, and can bar any person from entering a dangerous location. The rescue chief is in charge of providing entry to the site, and egress for the removal of victims when necessary. He is in charge of all rescue personnel. The chief EMS officer is in charge of patient care, triage, transportation, and all EMS personnel.

Whether the local chief executive working directly with the public safety chiefs is sufficient, or whether the executive needs a chief of operations under him, will vary depending on the structure of the public safety departments. *It is not implicit in the task that such an officer is necessary*. However, should one be appointed it is key that his function be coordinating and commanding operations, and not replacing line chiefs. Line command of each department should be left with the department's commanding officer.

Experience indicates that certain cautions are required when selecting an individual to be Chief of Operations. He must be someone who is acceptable to the other public safety chiefs, and who interacts with them and their departments on a regular basis. Should the fire chief, police chief, or other line officer be selected, he should not be required to fill both positions at the same time. For example, if the fire chief is selected as overall operations commander, the first deputy fire chief should take over line command of the fire department. The appointment of an overall commander must be made with a realistic scrutiny of the individual's experience and proven leadership ability.

Organization of authority and command *within* fire, police, and rescue departments is commonly well established and extremely reliable. Fire and police departments are structured in a paramilitary manner with a system of acknowledged rank and command. Rank is clearly visible on uniforms and turnout gear. Although sometimes a separate department, rescue is usually part of the fire or police department and works within the established command structure of that unit.

Mutual aid situations involving established procedures of call-up, communication, and command are common in the normal daily workings of fire, police, and rescue squads. Disciplined interaction between neighboring departments in these services rarely presents a problem in a mass casualty situation. Most regions acknowledge the local chief's command over any neighboring department he calls in to assist.

A pre-established organization is less common with EMS squads. Commonly, a clear understanding of rank and command among medical responders is *not* established. Even when it is, clear marking of rank for visual recognition rarely exists. It has been a common experience in many MCIs that either no EMS command was established, or a conflict arose.

Authority over EMS patient care operations in the field should belong to *the EMS squad that has primary, daily service responsibility for that area*. Only in rare cases should this authority be assigned to another group. The local EMS providers know the location and any special local problems. They also interface daily with fire, police, rescue, and hospital personnel.

EMS Command

In Mass Casualty Incidents, EMS command from any location other than the immediate disaster site will be detrimental to good patient care. Poor decisions will be made in the absence of necessary information. Conflicting orders will be given by field command personnel and headquarters. This will result in a lack of clear direction, leading to chaos. As with fire, police, and rescue command, the EMS authority must be at the site until the field is cleared of patients.

The attempt by a hospital to exercise command from its facility will cause decisions to be based on the hospital's priorities and not those at the site. This will be counterproductive to good triage and patient care. Since what is done in the field has the most critical impact on the ultimate survival rate, interference with field priorities will have an adverse effect on patient care and salvage.

Three EMS executives will be essential at the site. There must be an *overall* EMS chief who is in charge of all EMS operations in the field. Since the term *Chief* may be confusing, it is recommended that the term *Control* be used to designate the EMS executive who is in overall command.

The *Triage Officer* is in charge of sorting patients to establish priorities of treatment and transportation. He is also in charge of the care of patients awaiting transportation.

The *Transportation Officer* is in charge of all ambulances and directs the loading and transportation of patients. He is in continuous contact with the hospitals, and assures the balancing of the patient load among them. He acts as their liaison with the field. Experience has demonstrated the need for this position. When these tasks were included with those of the Triage Officer, it proved to be too broad an assignment for a single individual.

Several people who are normally readily available to respond should be trained for each of these functions. For each position there should be a clear ordering of those able to fill it, with a ranking such as *First Deputy Control, Second Deputy Control*, etc. This assures the availability of an individual for each position and avoids conflicts. It must be clear, however, that only *one* person fills the position at any one time.

The best means to allow easy identification of these officers in the field is the use of color-coded helmets. They are highly visible, and the possession of the *one* helmet that indicates a particular position makes confusion impossible.

These officers should, in most cases, be selected from the operations executives and training officers of the primary EMS provider. These officers have proven leadership ability within the squad and with other squads, and are known to the fire, police, and rescue officers. Their involvement in directing daily EMS activities is an important prerequisite. It is not uncommon to find the officer of training in the role of Control, and the chief executive of a service in the role of Triage Officer, or vice versa. The choice of service officers to fill these mass casualty positions should not be determined by an apparent similarity between the titles of their regular positions and the mass casualty positions. The choice should be based on individual skills, qualifications, and relationships. (At the onset of an incident, any EMT must be prepared to fill a command position until those designated to do so arrive.)

There are 2 approaches to command that, although apparently sensible in theory, will not work well and should not be considered viable alternatives.

1. Many plans have a team from the near hospital come to the site to take medical command. Under the best circumstances these teams function weakly; under the worst, not at all. This can result in a total breakdown in command. Few hospitals have sufficient personnel with command ability and MCI experience or training to assure that they will send only appropriate personnel. In many

hospitals such a team cannot be spared. Even when trained personnel are available, they, unlike local EMS executives, are unfamiliar with the personnel of the responding groups and do not interface daily with fire, rescue, and police officials. Lastly, when actual time trials are run, such hospital teams rarely reach the field in under 45 minutes from hospital alerting. Command in the first 45 minutes is critical.

2. Some regions develop mass casualty teams. In theory, regardless of the location of the MCI within the region, this team of experts is rushed in to take command of patient care. As efficient as this sounds, the reality is that such teams are almost inevitably too late in getting to the scene. Sometimes they can't get there at all. And, lastly, since they have not drilled and don't work with the personnel on a daily basis, they are not effective in spite of their expertise and experience.

In summary, appointing to command roles people who are not involved in the daily delivery of field EMS in that locality proves in almost every case to be unsuccessful and results in confusion, delay, and lack of compatible leadership.

Structure of the Communications System

Communication is often a serious problem in the conduct of a mass casualty response. Rarely, however, are difficulties caused by the kind of equipment used, or by a lack of equipment. Almost all fire departments have radio dispatch, and, often, tone activated call-up for volunteers or auxiliary personnel. There is vehicle-to-vehicle communication, and either direct or common dispatcher communication between neighboring fire departments. There are also a number of portable radios. Police departments generally have the same capabilities on different frequencies. Many EMS squads are associated with or dispatched by the fire or police service. They will have access to one of these radio networks.

Ambulances commonly have access to 2 separate radio frequencies. One is for dispatch and reaches either the fire or police department. The other is used for communication with the hospital in the delivery of daily emergency care. In many areas, a full range of EMS channels is available to all ambulances.

The fact that the radio traffic of each department is segregated from that of the others is a benefit in the disaster situation. Actually, it is essential because of the heavy radio traffic that occurs. This segregation helps avoid confusion. Since the fire chief's car, the police chief's car (or another police vehicle), and an ambulance will be stationed at the field command center, each of these separate radio systems can be monitored from this one location. Because this is done with equipment that is in daily use, it is not necessary to purchase, maintain, and bring to the site a separate mobile communications center.

With the current state of radio communications and the high output of today's mobile transmitters, any communications failure or auxiliary need can be handled with the use of vehicles operating on the same frequency. One vehicle can be positioned at the site and one at the other needed location. In the plan of one regional hospital, whenever a neighboring community has an incident, one police car from the town in which the hospital is located is placed at the entrance to the Emergency Department. Another is stationed at the field command center to provide a standby method of communication.

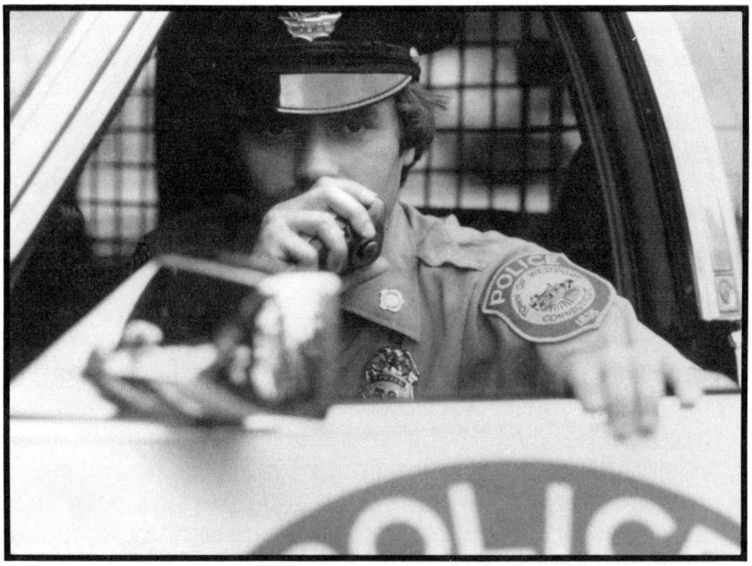

A unified emergency communications center that allows the handling of fire, rescue, police, and ambulance calls by one dispatcher, should provide for the rapid addition of personnel in its call-up system. Centers should be designed so that, during such a peak traffic load, one person can handle police traffic; one, fire and rescue; one, ambulance; and another, the telephone. If possible, jacks and switches should be provided to change from speakers to earphones to avoid confusion.

It is essential that all dispatchers have immediate access to the call-up plan. A good mass casualty plan and well-trained responders will be of no value if dispatchers don't know whom to call, how to bring in the needed personnel, and how to dispatch equipment. Up-to-date dispatch procedures written out in detail are a cornerstone of any successful plan.

LEVELS OF RESPONSE

It is common to find plans that divide the initial response into several levels. In these plans a level one, level 2, or level 3 response may be called for based on the incident that has occurred. This type of multilevel response is not recommended since initially not enough reliable information is available to make such a judgment. This approach also requires personnel to know several different plans. *One* basic response to any mass casualty situation, based on the need to handle 40 to 80 patients, is recommended. The public safety chiefs will have the ability to call in additional resources if necessary.

(A Mass Casualty Incident could be so unique or of such magnitude that even regional resources would be unable to deal with it. In that event, it might be necessary to call in state resources—the National Guard, for instance—or to have the scene declared a *disaster area*. Find out what steps are necessary for this procedure, and who should take those steps. It may be that the local chief executive should get in touch with State Police; it may be necessary to get in touch with the governor's office. Whatever actions are required, the procedure should be worked out in advance, and the details should be part of the response plan.)

Establishing Patient Priorities

The underlying principle that offsets the inability of regular resources to provide each patient with a normal level of care is *triage*. The use of triage saves the maximum number of lives possible—given the available time and resources. Patients are sorted into general categories and assigned priorities of treatment and transportation. A universal, international, color-coding and tagging system is used.

Red indicates top or first priority.

Yellow indicates second priority.

Green indicates nonserious, or third priority.

Black indicates the dead.

In normal daily care, *urgency* is the sole criteria. In mass casualty triage 2 factors determine priority: *urgency* and *potential for survival*. Because of this, patients in the second, or Yellow, priority are divided into 2 groups—Yellow and Yellow Prime. Yellow patients have been assigned a second priority because they can afford to wait. They are less urgent than Red priority patients. Yellow Prime patients have been assigned a second priority, even though they may need urgent care, because they are so grievously injured that they have little chance of survival. (Concepts and criteria of triage are discussed in further detail in Chapter 6.)

Triage relates to both priority of field care and priority of transportation. To deliver this care, an orderly method of organizing patients in the field is essential. Without it, triage will be ineffectual and may have little bearing on survival.

OPEN AND CLOSED INCIDENTS

Many Mass Casualty Incidents fit into a category described as *contained* or *closed*. A bus accident serves as a good example. The basic nature of a closed incident is that too many victims are confined in a small, undesirable place, usually filled with debris and wreckage. This makes careful evaluation and treatment in that location dangerous, if not impossible. This causes the need (after a minimum of stabilization) to evacuate the victims to a larger, safer place for re-evaluation, triage, and stabilization.

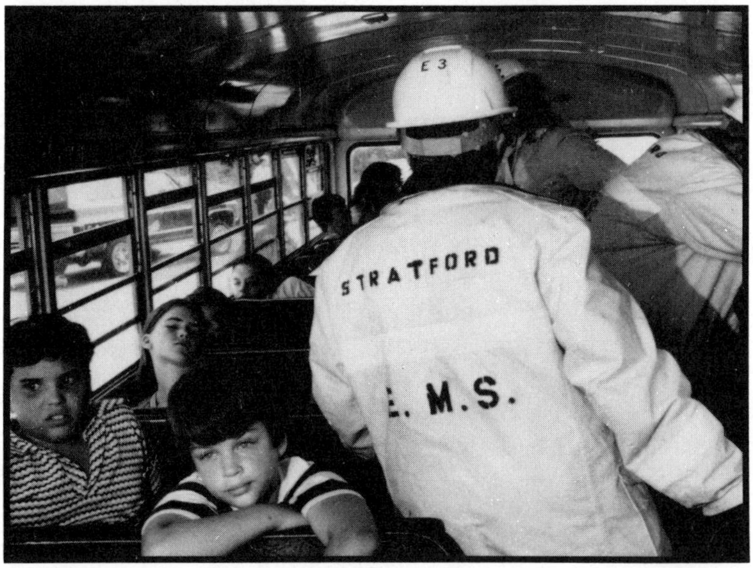

The other major category of Mass Casualty Incident is an *open* incident. An example would be a ferris wheel collapse in which victims are spread over a large area. The problems in this type of incident are the inverse of those in a closed incident. Here patients are too spread out to allow for proper care by the number of EMS responders that will be available. Although patients *can* be triaged and tagged where they lie, this proves to be problematic and ineffective. The Triage Officer moving throughout the field is too slow. Often when this is attempted, "haul and run" occurs from other parts of the field, or delay is inordinate. Furthermore, having patients of mixed priorities spread over a wide area makes retrieving patients of a given priority nearly impossible.

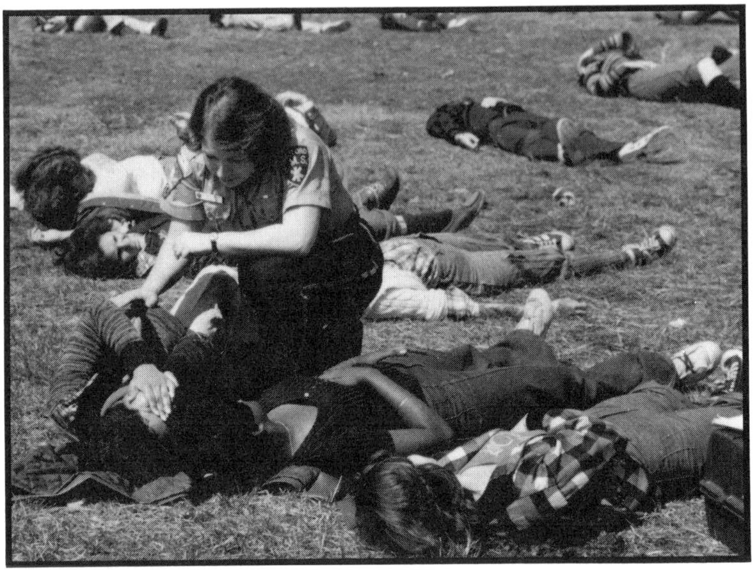

The problems of both closed and open incidents can be resolved by the establishment of a field triage and treatment center (which we will call the *patient collecting station*) near the victims and immediately accessible to incoming ambulances. In closed incidents, patients are rapidly stabilized, placed on appropriate immobilization devices, and then carried to the collecting station. Because of the nature of a closed incident, these patients are removed from the closed environment on the basis of space and accessibility, rather than medical priorities. It will often be necessary to remove several apparently less-seriously injured patients in order to gain access to those more seriously injured. As the patients arrive at the collecting station, they are given a priority by the Triage Officer or his deputy based on a quick visual evaluation. Patients are tagged and placed in rows or areas designated for each level of priority. These rows can be easily identified with colored flags. EMTs working at each location provide a more thorough survey, treat patients, and suggest reclassification as necessary.

In the open situation it is easier to bring patients to the collecting station in a sequence based on medical factors. While the actual assignment of priorities should be done by the Triage Officer, EMTs in the field can, with a rapid survey, locate those who appear to be Red and Yellow priorities, provide stabilization, and bring them to the collecting station using the appropriate rapid immobilization device.

All patients are brought to the collecting station. They are placed in clearly defined rows or areas based on the color-coded categories of priority. Patients are then transported to hospitals *from this location only*. In either closed or open situations, the practice of loading patients directly from where they lie into ambulances will become disorderly and will result in poor salvage.

Because all patients are placed in the central location, they can receive more care immediately as more EMTs arrive. Both the command module and the depository for extra supplies are located next to the collecting station.

The collecting station functions as a visually indentifiable center of activity. There is no question of where patients should be brought, or where ambulances should be sent. The patients are organized in identifiable areas based on their priority. This "ordering" is essential. Without this system, disorganized patient care and loss of triage priorities result.

Categories of Patients

In all of the Mass Casualty Incidents in our 22-incident study, over 99 percent of the patients were victims of trauma. The only variables were:

1. simple, localized injury;
2. multiple trauma;
3. smoke and/or superheated air and/or toxic fume inhalation; and
4. multiple trauma with smoke inhalation.

The difference between *simple, localized injury* and *multiple trauma* is really a matter of degree. Almost all incidents produce both levels of trauma. If ignition is involved, then patients with burns, and some suffering only from smoke inhalation, will be produced. Some trauma other than burns usually occurs at major fires, owing to falls, jumping, flying glass, collapse, and entrapment. However, at many fires the percentage of these patients compared to those suffering smoke inhalation can be extremely small. It is essential that the early reporting to hospitals include a clear statement of the mechanism and the type of structure, as well as the estimated scope.

Consider a report that says, "We have approximately 200 victims of a hotel fire," given at 2:00 AM. This should clearly alert everyone that, since the incident occurred at night with guests asleep in the hotel, there will be a high number of smoke-inhalation victims. From the report, "We have approximately 80 victims of a bus rollover," one should estimate a majority of MV trauma victims. Unless incidents are of a unique nature (such as chlorine leaks, group poisoning, etc.) the survivors are most likely to be *trauma victims*.

With the exception of building collapses and other forms of entrapment, or remote locations requiring "porter" carrying, the majority of patients should have arrived at the hospitals within a 2-hour period from the time of the response. Therefore, unless otherwise informed, hospitals should assume that their "share" of the patient number will arrive throughout a 2-hour period. The *clock* (or *rotary*)* system used to dispatch ambulances from the field will balance the incoming load over the time period and will maximize the time gap between arriving ambulances.

Because victims with multiple trauma represent the largest category of patients, a suitable device for transporting these victims must be used. The standard ambulance cot or canvas stretcher is inappropriate. (Many stores of old military stretchers exist. These are not only inappropriate but often unusable, due to deterioration.) Few pieces of special mass casualty equipment are really necessary. However, the availability of 100 to 120 simple wooden backboards is key. Since time pressures permit neither location of each injury, nor the excessive effort involved in immobilizing them, the boards can be used to reduce each patient to the normal anatomical position. The board effectively splints and supports all injuries, and stays with the patient both in the field and at the hospital.

*Ambulances are dispatched in sequence to hospitals 1, 2, 3, etc. When each hospital has been sent one ambulance, the rotation begins again.

Chapter 5

THE GENERAL PLAN: AN OVERVIEW

Anatomy of an MCI

In order to understand the implications of the material presented in the ensuing chapters, it is necessary to have an overview. The best way to obtain such an overview is to follow a sample MCI response in chronological order.

The mock incident we will use as our example is a school bus accident. It is witnessed by a resident who calls the local emergency dispatcher by CB radio, saying only that a school bus has crashed, giving the location, and adding, "There are lots of kids hurt, screaming, and bleeding."

The dispatcher immediately locates the mass casualty call-up in the emergency center's procedure book. The nearest police units are dispatched to the scene.* Then the fire department, rescue squad, and ambulance crews are activated, in that sequence, by use of the normal tone-alert call-up system. Using the telephone or, preferably, pagers, key disaster-response EMS personnel are then contacted.

The radio messages are short, precise, and exactly as they appear in the guidebook.

"Police Units 20 and 40 respond to an unconfirmed signal '1000' at Smithtown Highway between Exits 4 and 5, north lane."

"KDT 130 to all Trumbull firemen and rescue personnel with a signal '1000.' All fire and rescue personnel report to your firehouses."

"KDT 130 to all Trumbull ambulance personnel with a signal '1000.' All ambulance personnel report with turnout gear, crash kits, and tone-alert receivers to headquarters."

"KDT 130 to mass casualty officers with an *unconfirmed* signal '1000' at Smithtown Highway between Exits 4 and 5, north lane—a bus accident."

Fire and rescue trucks depart as soon as enough personnel are available. The on-duty first call ambulance also leaves.

Vehicles sign on the air so the fire chief and other key personnel can hear when units are manned and leaving. But *no acknowledgement* is transmitted by the dispatcher.

The dispatcher next notifies the near hospitals that an as yet unconfirmed mass casualty disaster is in progress.

Next, back-up dispatchers are called in. The town's chief executive and others on the official call-up list are notified. Included on this list should be a tow truck operator, some school bus drivers, and town hall personnel.

*In most towns, police units can get to the scene faster than fire equipment. In rural areas where local fire departments may be closer than the highway patrol, the dispatch sequence should be fire before police. The preplanning criterion is, whoever can get there faster.

At the scene of the incident, the first uniformed responder to arrive, usually a police officer, assesses the traffic situation and places his car as a barrier to oncoming traffic.

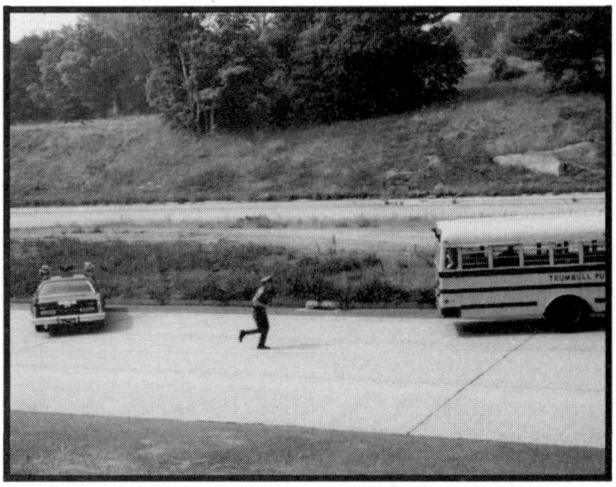

He boards the bus and speaks to the injured to reassure and calm them. He shows them how to apply direct pressure to bleeding wounds and tells them that assistance is on the way. During this time, he estimates the maximum number of injured.

If there is any chance of fire, explosion, or other immediate danger, he rapidly begins to move people off the bus—regardless of their injuries. In a case such as this, many of the less-severely injured will probably have begun to leave the bus before his arrival, either on their own or with the help of passers-by.

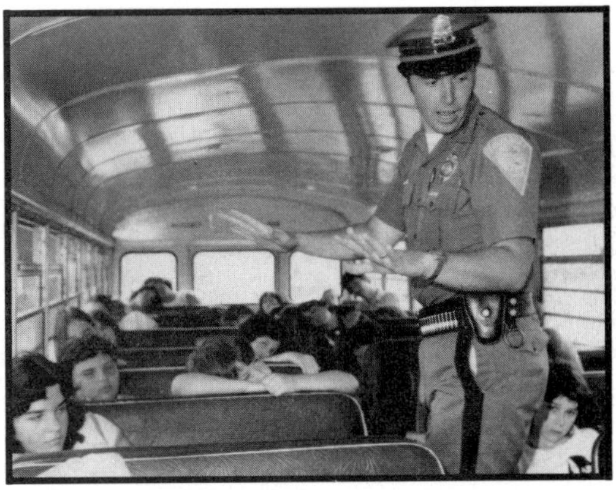

If the bus appears safe, the police officer does not evacuate the injured from it.

Next, the police officer radios headquarters with a short, simple message confirming the signal "1000," and estimating the number of victims. He also gives the exact location and best routes of approach.

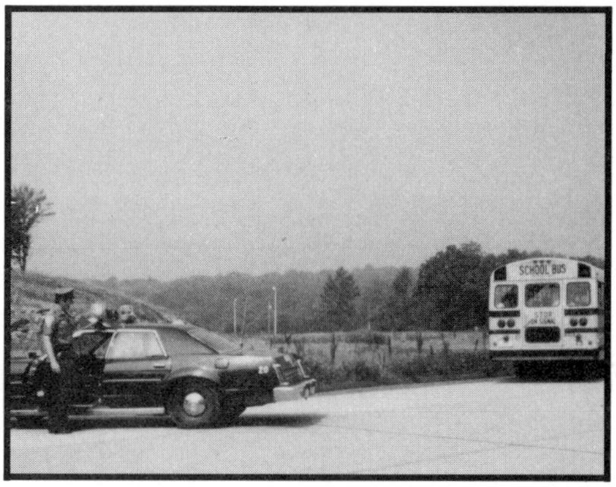

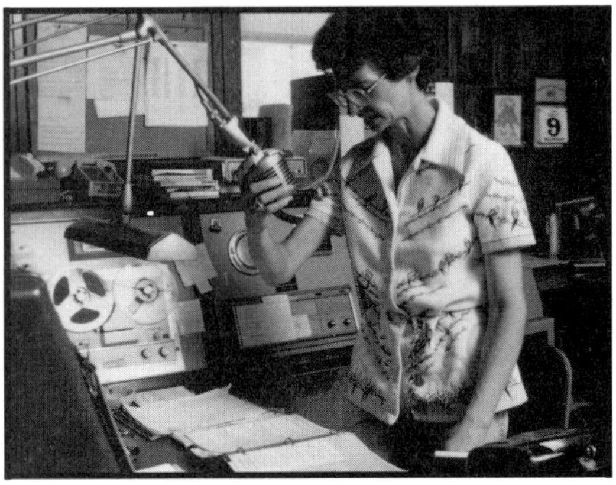

On each frequency—fire, police, and ambulance—the confirmation of the signal "1000" is transmitted, along with the exact location and routing instructions. From this point forward, to avoid confusion, no coded messages are used. All transmissions should be short, precise, and in clear, normal language.

At the communications center, the pre-established procedures are continued upon confirmation of the MCI. A full region-wide response is rapidly activated.

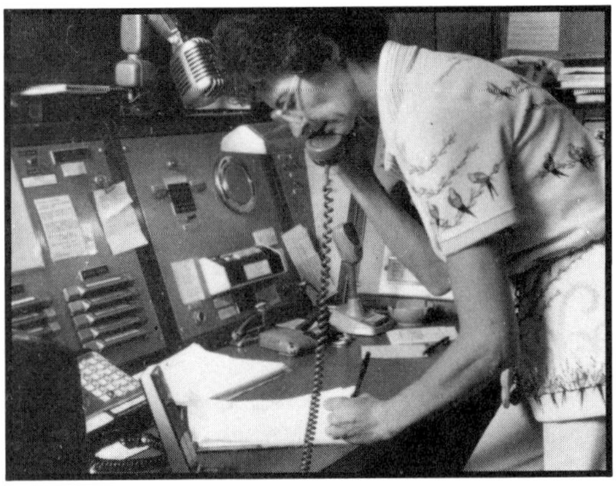

The near hospitals are informed that a *confirmed* mass casualty incident is in progress, and are given the estimated number of injuries—in this case, 60. Any hospitals that have not yet activated their disaster plans do so at this time.

The EMS squads and 10 to 12 ambulances on the call-up list are told to respond with mass casualty equipment and double crews. At least one, and possibly more, volunteer EMS services from within the region have been predesignated to respond with "all members" to provide a substantial force of EMTs at the scene. Neighboring police and fire departments are contacted as specified in the plan.

The first fire officer at the scene determines the fireground problems and evaluates the safety of the scene. He then locates his fire lines of defense and confers with the police officer on the best location for incoming units. The police officer will guide the incoming equipment as it arrives. Note that a fire truck will be positioned to control each end, and the rescue truck will be placed as close as is safe to minimize hauling of equipment.

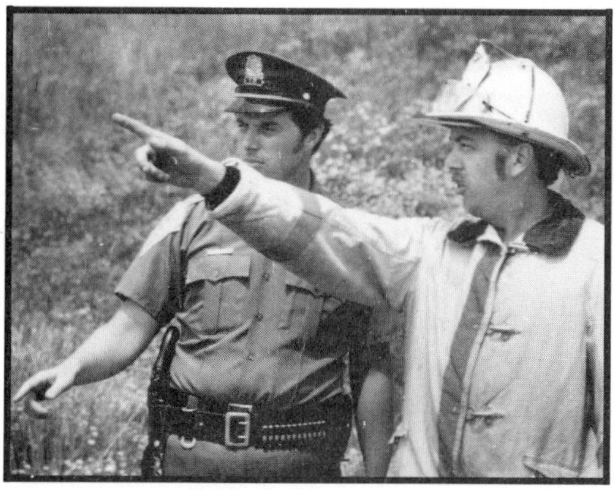

As fire and rescue personnel arrive, they are briefed by the senior fire officer on the scene, who indicates that the area is safe for personnel to proceed. Fire and rescue units are placed and fire lines are charged.

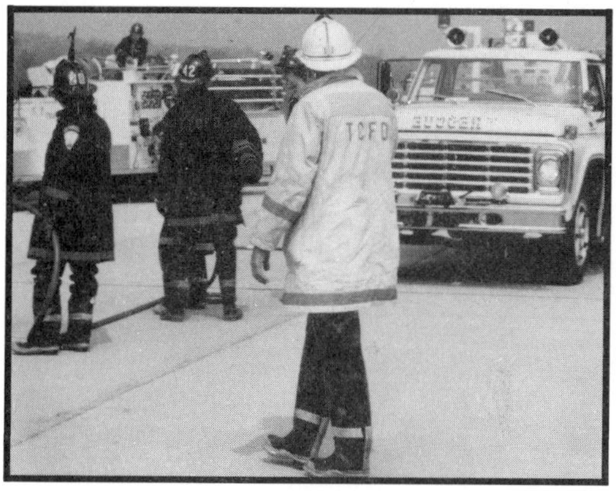

Rescue personnel shore and cable the damaged school bus as necessary, and unload their equipment.

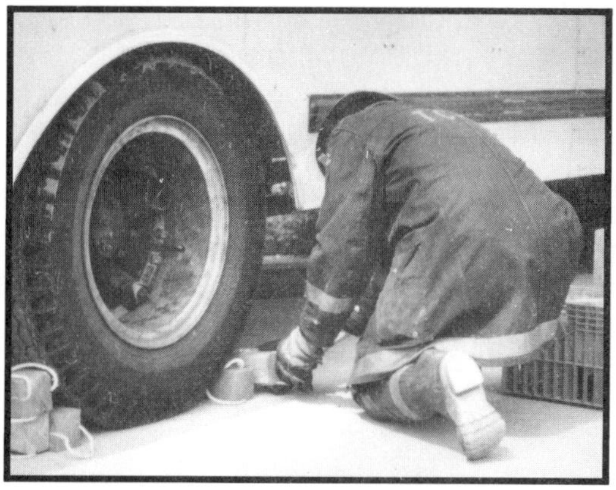

When the bus is secure, fire and rescue personnel enter.

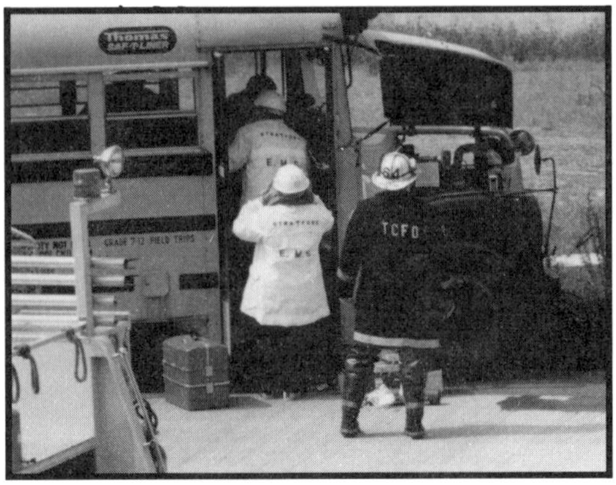

The on-call ambulance arrives and is directed to its proper position at a safe distance from the bus. This ambulance, with its direct radio contact with the near hospitals, will serve as the command module and as a field surgical center, if necessary.

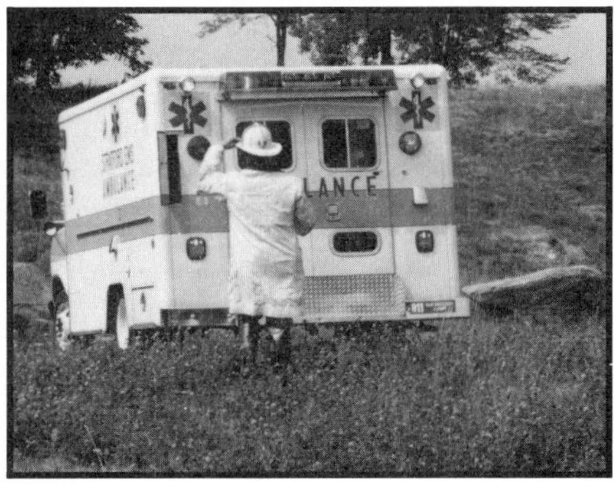

Its crew take their carry-in equipment and enter the bus. Working with the fire and rescue responders and EMTs, they move rapidly from one patient to the next, ensuring that hemorrhage is stopped and that each victim has a patent airway and adequate ventilation. Until *all* victims have been checked to this extent, no other individual patient care is started.

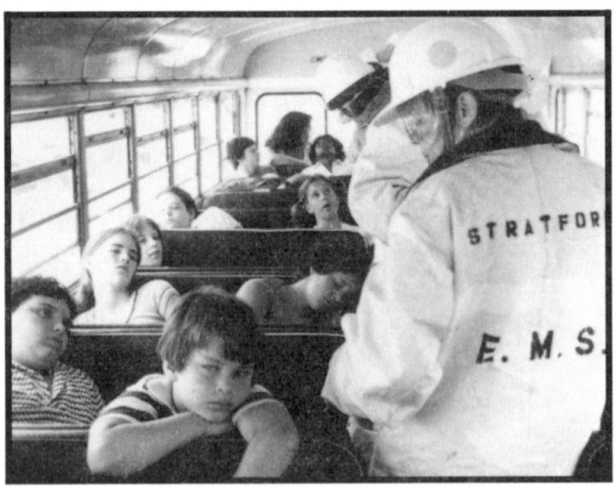

Under the direction of a bus commander (a crew member of the command module ambulance), further stabilization is then provided. No time-consuming treatment is started on grievously injured patients at this time.

A fire or rescue officer is positioned at each entrance to assist when needed and to keep unnecessary personnel off the bus. If there are egress problems, the rescue team sets up tools and cuts a suitable egress route. The fire chief continues to survey the scene to be certain it remains safe.

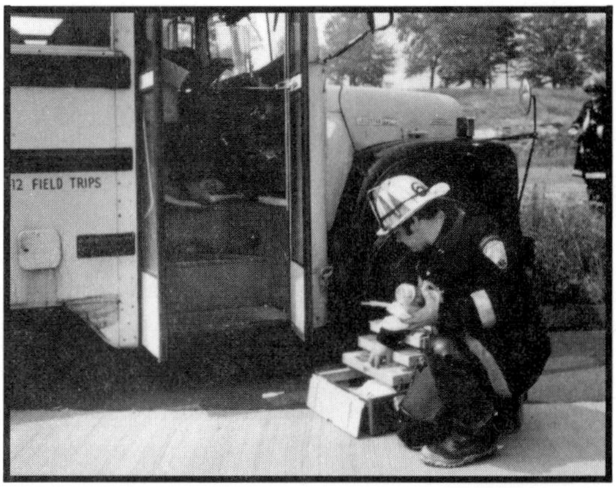

Outside the bus several activities are now taking place simultaneously. Salvage covers are laid out to create a patient-collecting and triage station near, but at a safe distance from the bus. It is important for patient safety that this location be at a slightly higher elevation than the bus, to avoid possible runoff of gasoline or extinguishing foam.

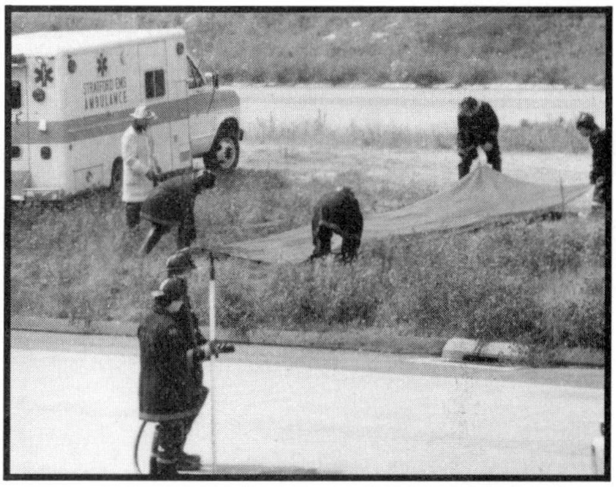

When the chief EMS officer arrives, he is quickly briefed by the EMT acting as EMS commander (the crew chief of the first-call ambulance) and by the fire chief. He then takes over the role of Control (chief of EMS field operations), coordinating all EMS activities from the command module. He informs each near hospital about the scope of the situation, the general nature of the injuries, and what it can expect to receive (that is, the proportion of the casualty load he anticipates directing to that hospital. For instance, 2 near hospitals may each receive ½ of the total.)

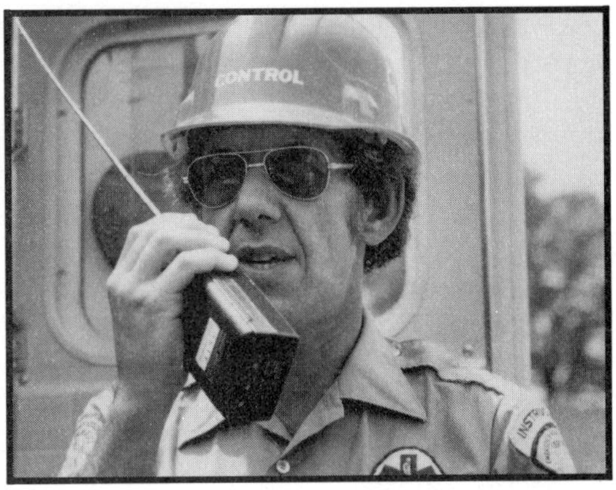

When the police chief arrives, he checks the deployment of his personnel and makes adjustments if he feels it is necessary. He then takes his position at the command module. He confers with Control on the roads and routing to be used. Incoming police report to the command module and receive instructions from the chief or his alternate.

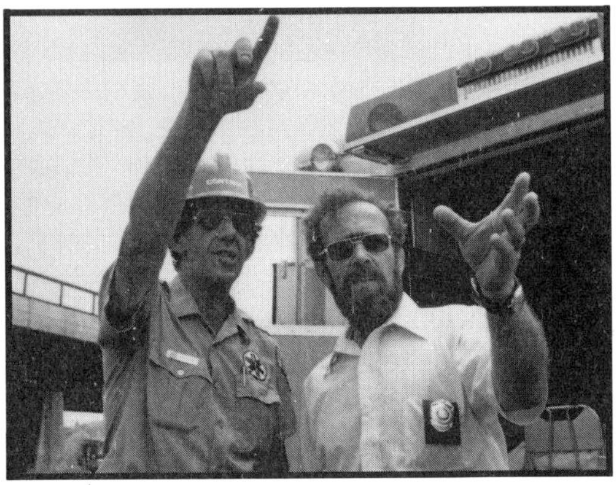

As additional fire equipment arrives, one truck is placed at the patient-collecting station, between it and the bus, to create a protective barrier and line of defense in case of fire.

All incoming ambulances are directed to the loading area which has been established near the collecting station. Crew members report to the Transportation Officer for specific assignments.

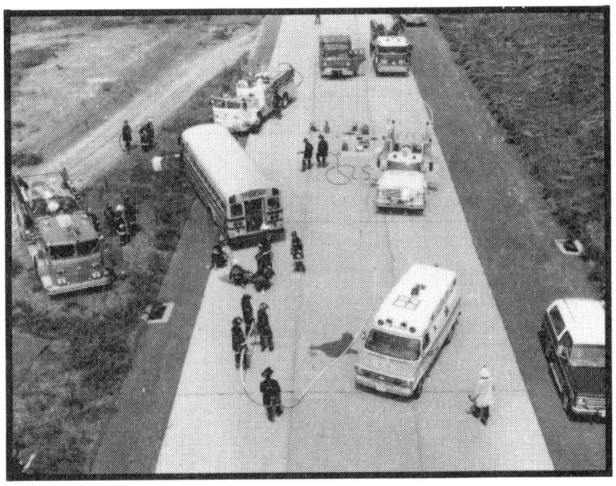

As additional mass casualty equipment arrives, it is down-loaded—immobilization boards near the bus, and medical supplies at the command module. Equipment in each category (cervical collars, bandages, portable oxygen, etc.) is placed in orderly piles. The special mass casualty supply trunks are placed at the collecting station, and color-coded triage flags are set up. Patients, when triaged, will be placed in rows by the appropriately colored flags.

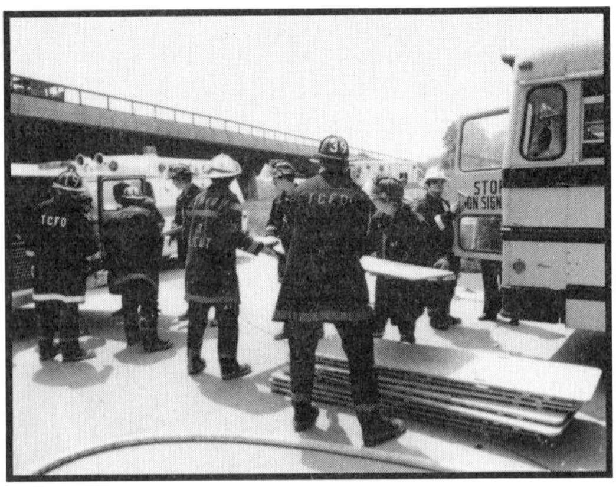

Additional fire and police units arrive at the site from neighboring towns. But even with county and state police responding, there are rarely enough police to direct traffic, keep routing open, and maintain crowd control. Fire personnel using hoses or ropes can be used to form efficient crowd lines, backed by police officers who patrol the perimeter established by the firemen.

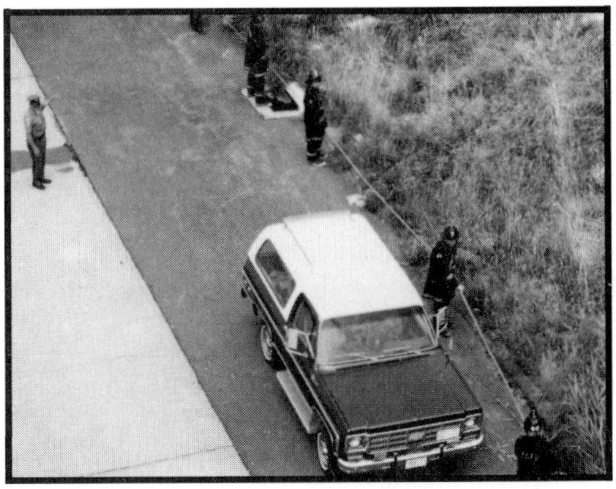

Depending on travel time, it is now 10 to 15 minutes from the first alarm and phase one has been completed. Fire defense is established. All patients have had a primary survey. Patients are being stabilized and treated as they lie. A command post is functioning. Four or 5 ambulances are present. Proper immobilization equipment is ready. A suitable collecting and treatment station has been established. Fifteen to 25 EMTs are present.

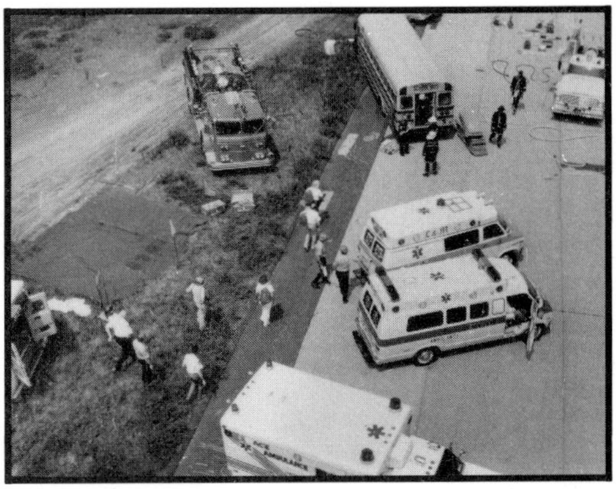

Had there been a serious threat of ignition, patients would have been taken off the bus in any way possible, regardless of their injuries. In the absence of that threat, they have been rapidly stabilized on the bus. No full survey or more involved care has been started. Because of the number of patients and the limited number of EMTs that can work in the space of the bus, it will require great skill to achieve even this stabilization in the first 10 to 15 minutes.

From this point, there should be no delay in moving the patients to the collecting station for further evaluation, triage, further treatment, and transportation on a priority basis to the near hospitals. Patients come off the bus in a sequence dictated by space and location problems, not on the basis of priority.

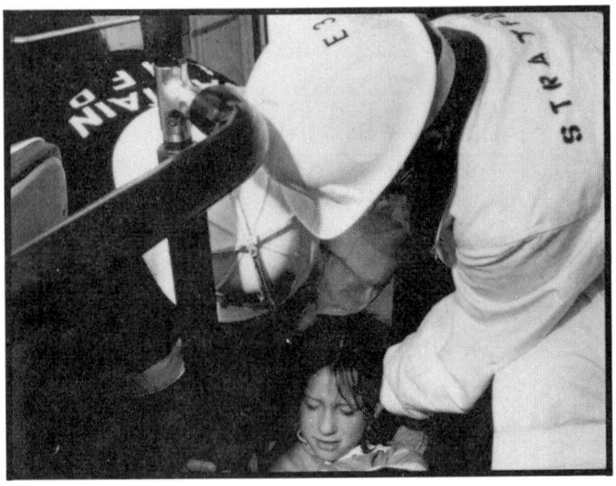

Each seriously injured patient is quickly stabilized on a backboard, split litter, or long board. Rigid boards provide stabilization and support to all parts of the body, so no time need be spent splinting individual injuries.

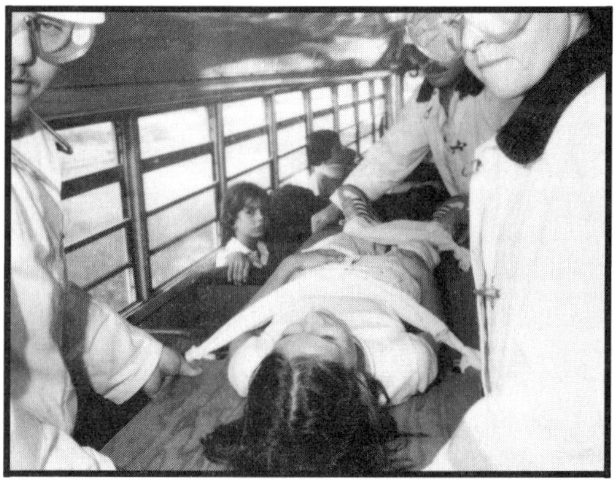

Once the aisle is cleared of patients, any ambulatory non-severe patients are helped out to provide more workspace on the bus.

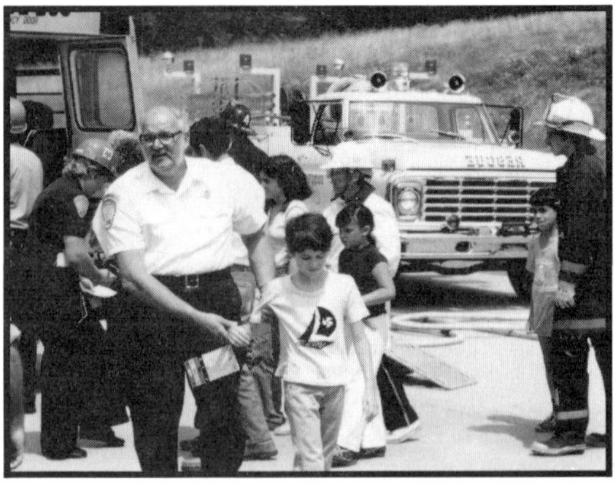

The first medical triage is performed as the patients arrive at the collecting station. This is always the case in an open situation where patients are spread over a wide area. However, in a closed situation the option does exist to do the initial triage as the patients emerge from contained areas (such as when they come off the school bus). Immediately after each patient leaves the bus he can be rapidly evaluated, assigned a priority color, and tagged with an identification number and color by the Triage Officer or his deputy.

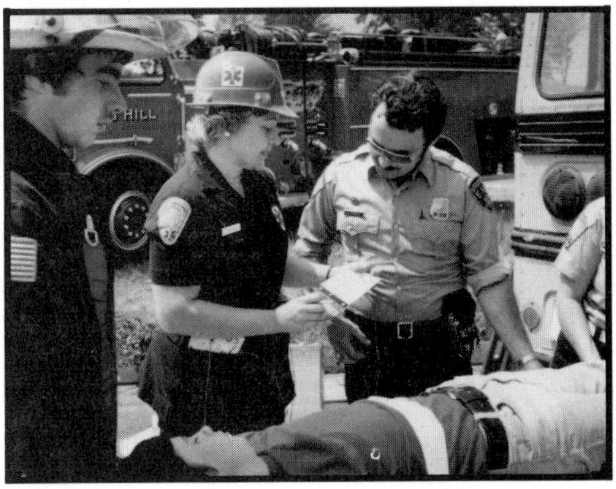

At the collecting station, the patients are placed in rows which clearly separate them by priority color. If the Triage Officer has been assigning priorities at any other location, he returns to the collecting station when a group of patients begin to mass there. Under his direction, groups of EMTs treat patients more thoroughly. Based upon the more detailed survey or on a deterioration in a patient's condition, patients are reclassified, retagged, and moved to higher priority rows.

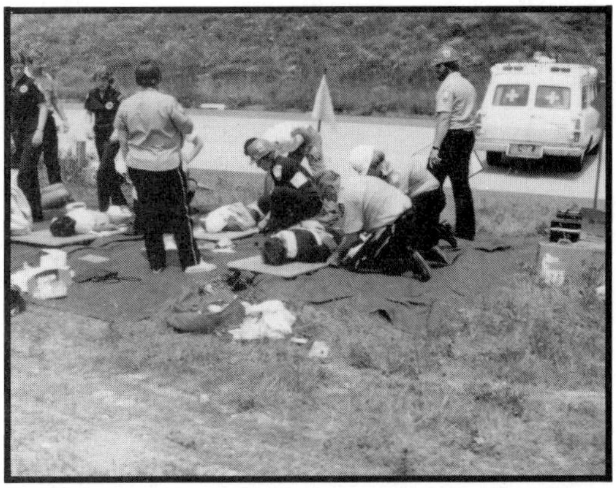

The prime responsibility of the Triage Officer at this point is to direct patient care at the collecting station, and to determine priorities within the Red row. His deputy is now doing the initial tagging. The Triage Officer must consult with EMTs who feel a patient should be moved to a higher priority row. And it is essential that he stay in constant communication with the Transport Officer at all times.

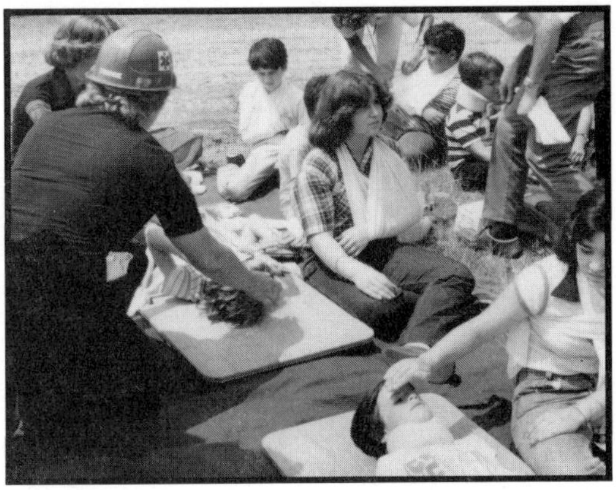

Under the direction of the Transportation Officer, Red category patients are loaded 2 to an ambulance. The officer quickly notes the identification number, condition, and injuries of each. He tells the driver which hospital to go to and gives clear routing instructions.

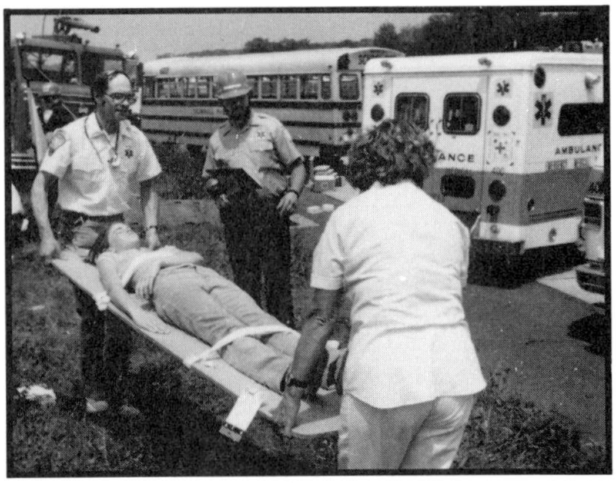

It is essential that nonlocal drivers have explicit directions so that they won't get lost. (Marked maps are suggested if routing is complex.)

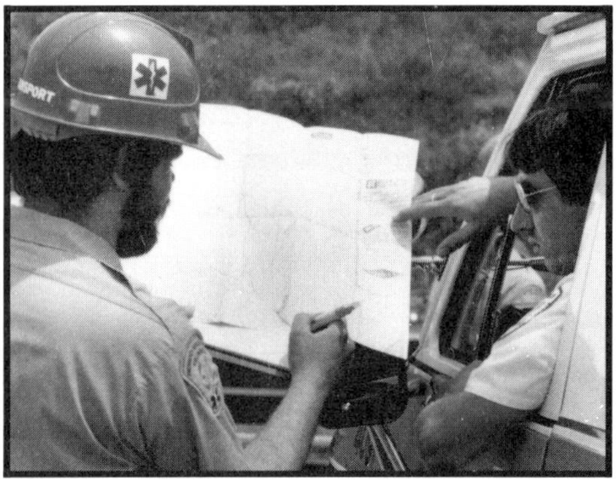

The Transportation Officer then contacts the hospital and tells them which ambulance is en route and what the conditions and injuries of the patients are. During a Mass Casualty Incident, communication between each individual ambulance and the hospital would clutter the frequency; it is not necessary unless an emergency develops en route.

If more than one near hospital is to be used, ambulances are dispatched in alternating turns to each (a *clock* system).

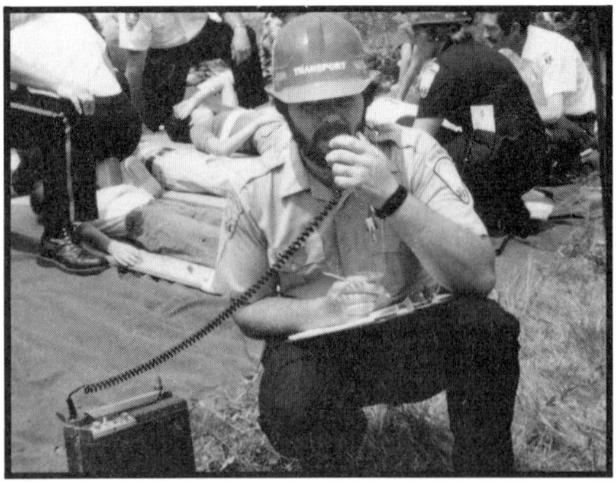

Control is moving from place to place, deploying personnel as necessary and directing all EMS operations. If he has to stop to fill any specific function, he should not be committed for long. To ensure contact between the command module and Control, a runner is present at the command module who is always aware of Control's location. If Control is needed and the runner is unable to locate him, the runner should radio the dispatcher who activates Control's pager. At this signal, Control should immediately return to the command module.

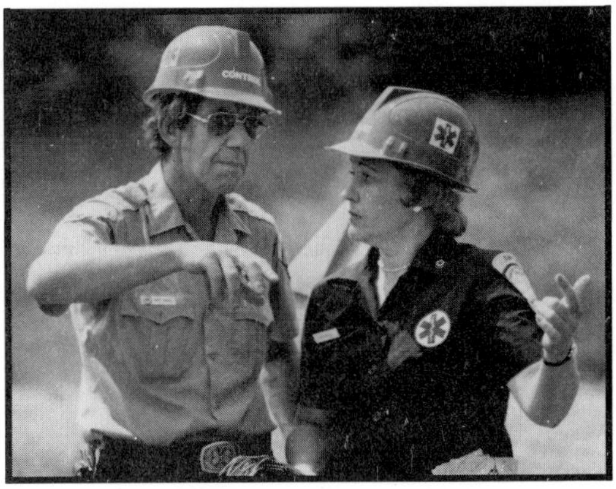

At this point, all the ambulances that were summoned have arrived. EMS operations are now composed of 4 elements.

1. Care, stabilization, and immobilization of those patients still on the bus
2. Moving patients to the collecting station, categorizing and tagging them, and placing them in the appropriate rows
3. Caring for patients at the collecting station and reclassifying them when necessary
4. Loading and transporting the highest priority patients

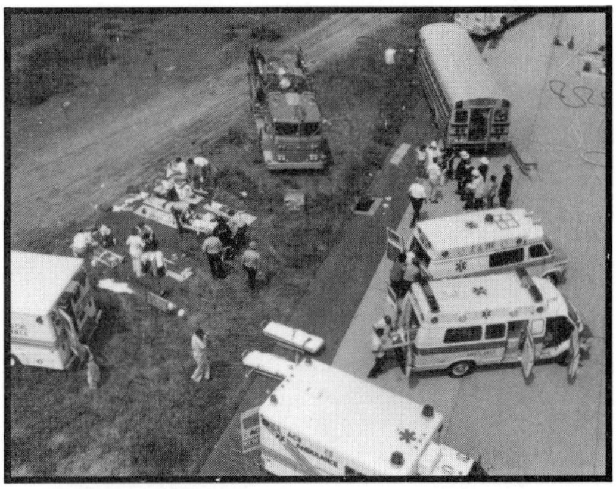

A specific officer is in charge of each of these functions. Once assigned to a certain task, each EMT should continue it and not move to any other unless directly ordered to do so by an EMS executive.

As few patients remain on the bus, the bus commander orders some personnel to leave and report to Control for reassignment. If Control is unavailable, EMTs should report to the collecting station to receive assignments from the Triage Officer or the Transport Officer. The collecting station is now the place where the most help is needed, and the additional EMTs will provide better individual patient care.

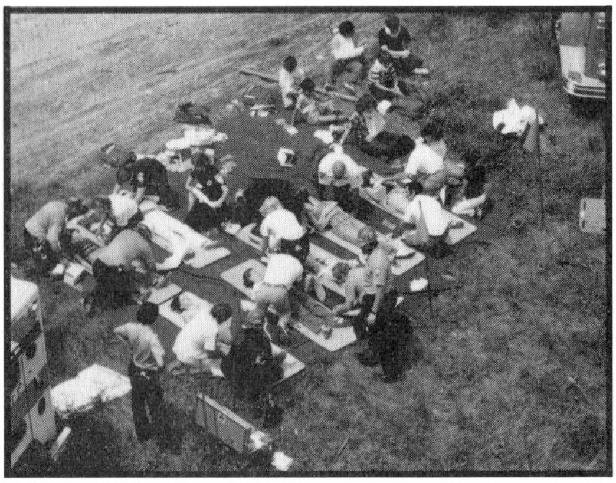

While these EMS procedures are being carried out, many other situations develop at the site. The chief executive of the town arrives and confers with Control and the fire, police, and rescue chiefs. While direct line control remains with them, the chief executive brings in needed support, solves problems, and has overall authority.

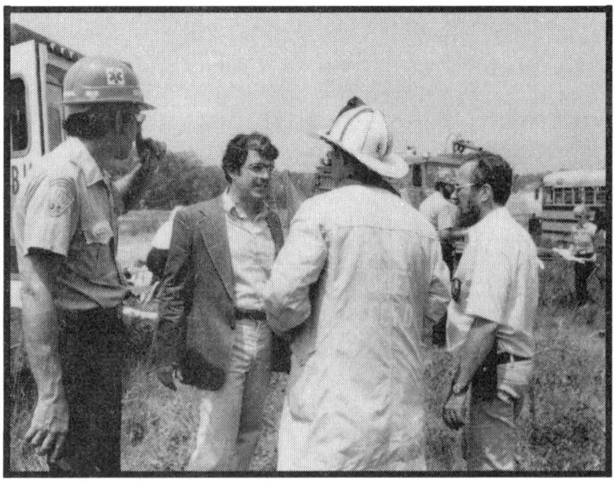

Key town hall staff have been summoned to their offices, day or night. Under the direction of the chief executive's deputy, the town hall gives out information, works with neighboring towns, locates needed items, and handles any other necessary tasks. For instance, if it appears that field operations will continue for a long time, town hall arranges to have food brought in. Representatives of the local government are sent to the nearest hospitals to help with identification, deal with relatives of the victims, and fill any other needs that arise.

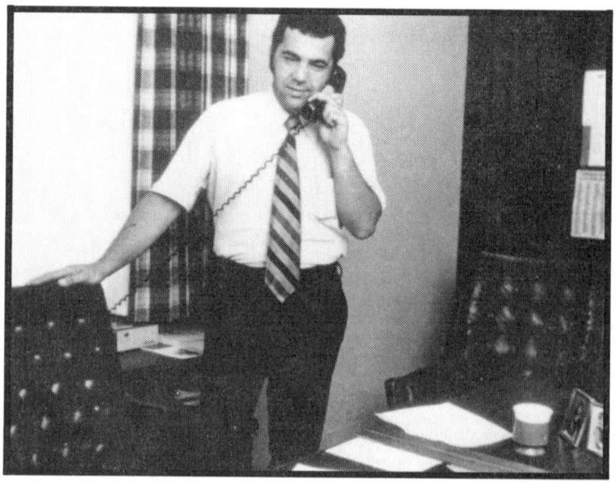

When advanced medical personnel arrive, such as physicians, IV nurses, paramedics, and other ALS personnel, their attention is directed to patient stabilization and care at the collecting station. In many cases, a hospital medical team will not arrive at the site in under 45 minutes. When such a team does arrive, it should not take over administration of the field. Working with the Triage Officer, it should perform the task it and it alone can do: providing a higher level of medical care to those remaining in the field.

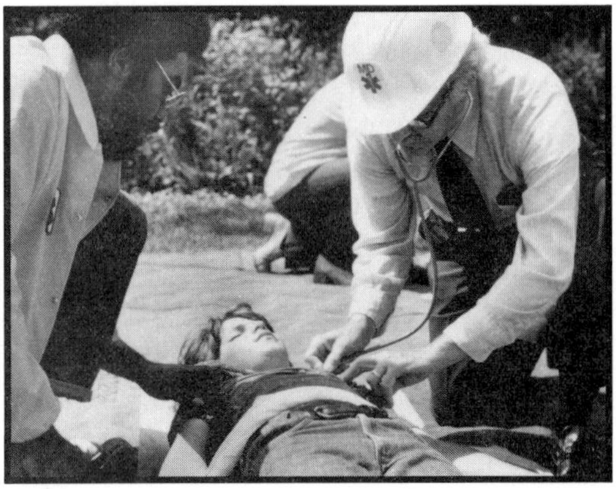

It is now betwen 45 and 60 minutes from the time of the alarm. All Red priority patients have been cleared and transportation of Yellow priority patients has begun.

At this point, many people have been working furiously for a prolonged period. The operation seems to be going on and on, and the initial response to the challenge is wearing thin. Physical exhaustion begins to set in.

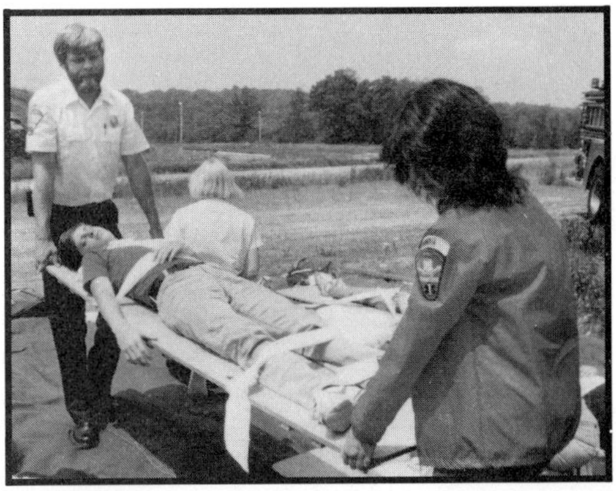

For some individuals, the emotional strain may become intolerable. Even a highly trained EMT may "come apart at the seams." This is where good leadership is essential. If a responder has just become a victim, he must be removed from the field gracefully without tying up other personnel. He should be assigned to the next ambulance leaving for the hospital.

Anyone—responder or patient—who becomes hysterical in the field will be extremely disruptive to the

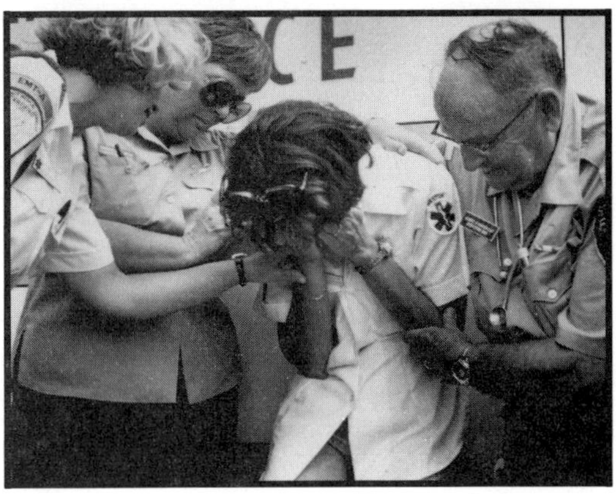

operation. Regardless of a patient's medical needs, if he becomes hysterical he should be removed to the hospital on a high priority. Pragmatism must override justice for the sake of order in the field.

Should any responder become seriously ill or injured, he too should be treated immediately, regardless of other more urgent priorities. This will keep his fellow responders functioning and maintain order and discipline.

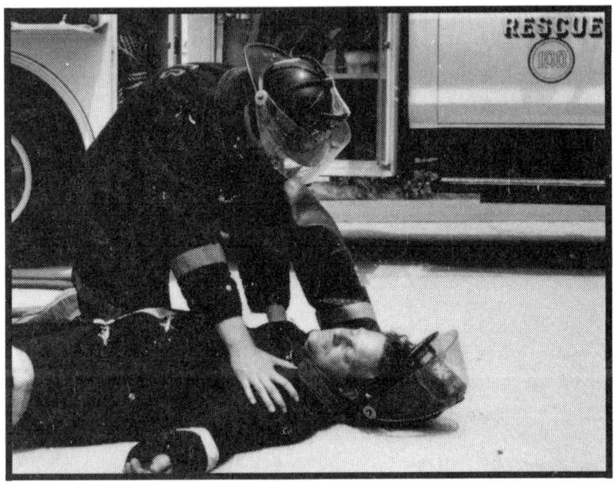

Finally, only Green priority patients remain. Some ambulatory Green patients may have been transported earlier as "extra" sitting patients in ambulances carrying those of higher priority. Nonambulatory Green patients are now transported, 2 at a time, by ambulance.

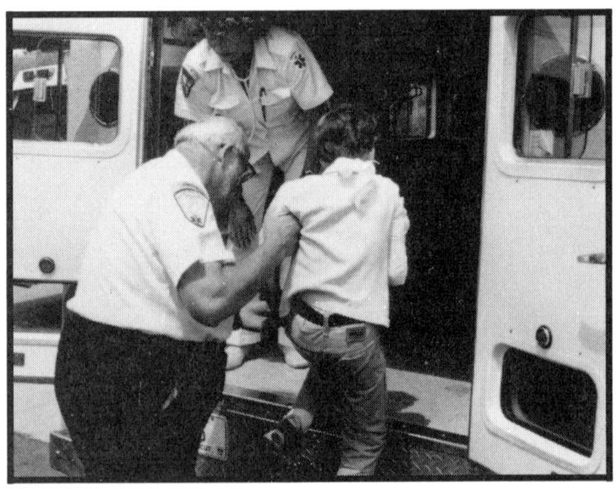

When all that remain are Green priority patients who are capable of walking, they are loaded onto a bus brought to the site for this purpose. When the bus is about to leave, Control consults with the near hospital to determine whether or not the bus will "leapfrog" to an outlying hospital that has little or no load. Departure time and estimated arrival time are then confirmed with the receiving hospital.

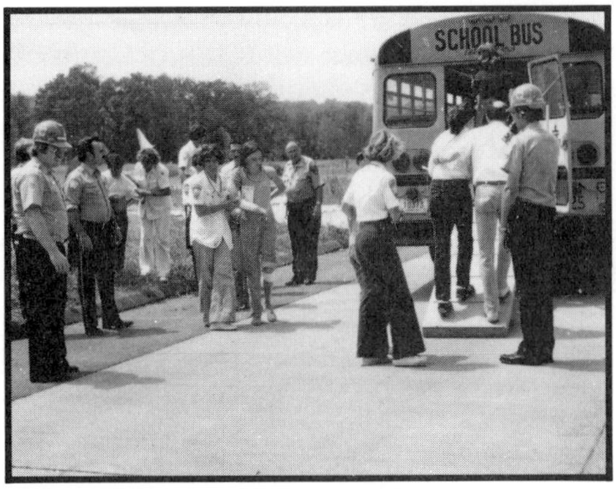

Five to 8 EMTs with portable oxygen, suction, crash kits, and a portable radio travel aboard the bus. A fully equipped and crewed ambulance leads it at a reasonable speed. Should a patient deteriorate suddenly en route, the ambulance will provide several options for that patient's care.

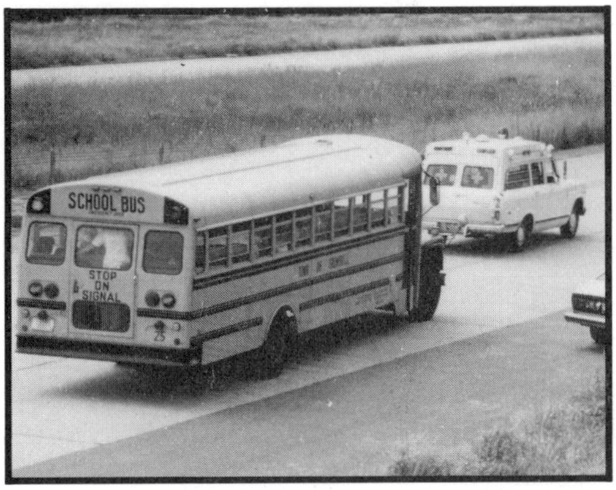

When the field is cleared of patients, all ambulances and EMTs go to the near hospitals and assist the staff in caring for patients and in transporting patients to other hospitals.

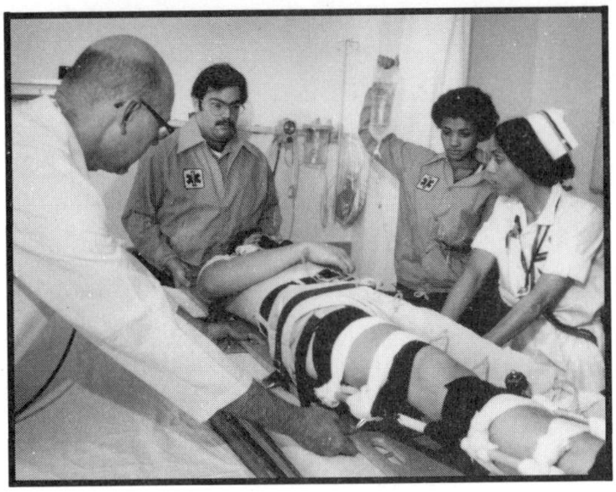

Summary of the Incident

A brief summary will show that this method of response has achieved the primary goals of dealing with any mass casualty situation. A citizen contacted the dispatch center, which activated the proper local response. The pre-established plan provided for the orderly summoning of the correct resources to the site. In the first few minutes, when only a few EMTs were available, any patient who could be saved by a simple maneuver, such as repositioning the head to provide an airway or applying direct pressure to stop bleeding, received that treatment. Only when *all* patients had been checked and treated at this level, did individual patients receive more stabilization and care.

All multitrauma patients were placed on boards which supported and splinted all of their bones and joints. Their wounds were supported and immobilized. They were then quickly removed from the limiting environment of the bus.

Without delay or a detailed, time-consuming examination, patients were assigned a priority and placed at the collecting station in rows by priority in an organized manner. Here they received the maximum care possible based on the number of available EMTs, and were evaluated carefully. Where indicated, they were moved into a higher priority. The most urgent and salvageable were transported first, as ambulances became available. Patients were sent to the near hospitals using a clock method of distribution that ensured a balanced load.

When advanced medical personnel began to arrive, the physical organization of the field made it easy for them to locate the patients *most in need of their help*.

Organization, discipline, command, and communication existed from beginning to end. This prevented many problems from developing, and provided the machinery for remediating the real problems inherent in the incident.

The plan automatically summoned all EMTs from tone-dispatched volunteer EMS services, and similarly summoned extra neighboring volunteer fire personnel. This ensured the presence of a large group of EMTs to augment the ambulance crews that were called, providing against any short-fall that may have occurred.

No mass casualty response can meet all the needs of every patient. No single plan can incorporate solutions to all the specific problems that might arise in the many different kinds of possible incidents. The structure of the response presented here is simple. It can be easily learned by all involved. This plan does not ensure normal, daily levels of care to each patient, but it does provide the best care possible with the limited resources that will be available, and it focuses on maximizing the number of survivors.

Chapter 6

MASS CASUALTY TRIAGE

Triage: An Overview

Before going into the details of the mass casualty triage system, it is important to discuss 2 concepts upon which the system is based.

Too frequently in MCIs the patients first removed from the field are those who are nearest to the arriving ambulances, those who are the earliest to be extricated, or those who are the most gravely injured. Although exact records regarding patient care sequence are rarely available, interviews with hospital Emergency Department personnel clearly confirm that the dead and the catastrophically injured are commonly in the first groups to arrive. Since a high percentage of these patients do not survive, undue resources have been directed to patients who are the least salvageable, while other patients who are more salvageable receive little or no attention.

When catastrophically injured patients with poor salvageability are the first to be transported, a further misapplication of resources occurs at the near hospitals. These patients require labor-intensive care, often including time-consuming surgery, to stabilize vital functions. Therefore, they commonly tie up available Emergency Department or Operating Room personnel for hours, effectively taking the near hospital out of commission. This results in either the overloading of another near hospital, or dangerously long transit times to an outlying facility for critical patients with better salvage potential.

By definition, in an MCI, resources do not allow for the meeting of all patients' needs within the necessary time frames. Therefore, a system of triage is used to sequence patient care. The term *triage* comes from the French and means "to sort" or "to categorize."

Depending upon the situation, there are varying criteria for sorting. In the daily delivery of emergency care, life-threatening urgency is the sole criterion. It is the basis for the sequence of survey and assessment. Similarly, in the properly run Emergency Department, patients are seen on the basis of urgency—not in the order they arrived.

Establishing priority in MCIs also involves urgency as the first sorting criterion. Patients are either *urgent* or *not urgent*. However, a substantial change from daily EMS criteria next occurs in determining *which* of the very urgent will be given priority. In daily EMS it is the most urgent injured who receive resuscitative care first. In a mass casualty situation the next criterion for establishing priority among the very urgent must be *potential for survival*. This consideration is alien to our daily experience and must be carefully ingrained in the mass casualty training of all EMS personnel. It must be stressed that the criteria used daily by EMS personnel *are inappropriate in MCIs*. If the most grievously injured, the clinically dead, the moribund receive resuscitative efforts, the overall survival rate will suffer.

Another key change in the hospital emergency medical treatment during an MCI, is separation of the concepts of *stabilization* and *definitive treatment*. *All* patients must be stabilized before further care is given to any individual. (In some surgical cases this distinction may not be possible. However, in most patients a fairly clear distinction between stabilization, reparation, and definitive care can be readily made.) Only after *all* patients are stabilized and additional patients are not forthcoming should definitive care become the focus of medical personnel. Again, the idea of not "completely" treating a patient being cared for is alien to traditional medical concepts and will take some rethinking and retraining.

An MCI patient will be triaged many times, both in the field and in the hospital. Frequency will depend upon such factors as the amount of elapsed time (allowing for patient deterioration), availability of time or resources for more definitive patient assessment, and availability of a wider range of diagnostic ability and equipment in the receiving hospital. Before discussing these points, it is important to review the concepts and methods of field triage.

Field Triage Concepts

Triage in the field involves priorities both for transportation to the hospital and for care in the field. Triage doesn't work in the field unless patients are tagged. Without the aid of a visible reminder, it

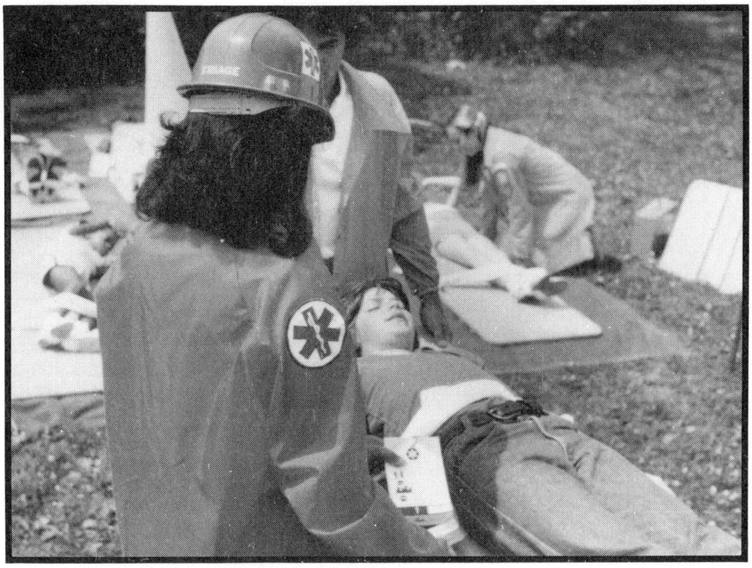

is impossible to keep track of earlier decisions. Tagging alone, however, will not do the job. The tagged patients must be placed in rows by priority at the collecting station. Since each tagged patient is placed upon a rigid board, moving the patients will not be injurious.

Under an international convention, color codes are used to indicate priority:

Red—most urgent
Yellow—second priority
Green—third priority
Black—dead

Although the use of only 4 colors may present problems, another system of colors or numbers should not be instituted. The convention assures that personnel from any location will be familiar with the code.

Three types of tags are available. The most common and inexpensive type contains a series of tear-off segments. There is one

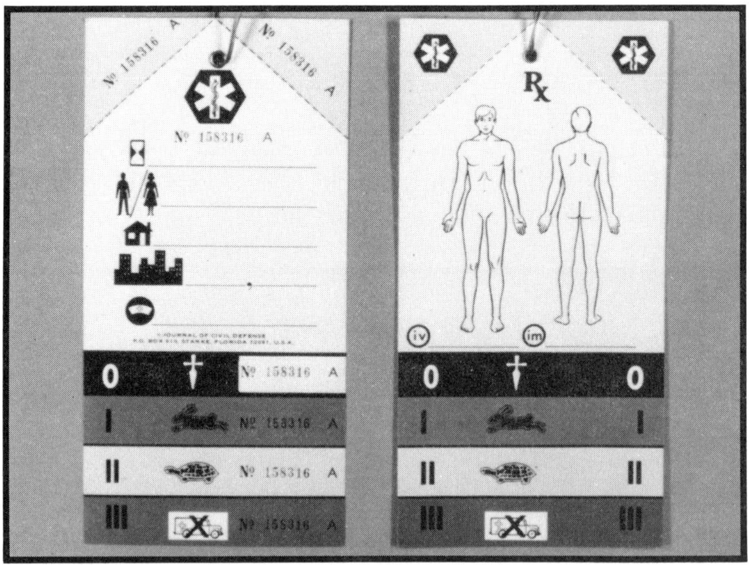

tear-off segment for each color, sequenced from least urgent (green on the outside) to most urgent (red on the inside), followed by black. The tag is placed on the patient, and his urgency is noted by the outermost color. Should a patient deteriorate and become more urgent, the EMT can raise the patient's priority by tearing off an additional segment. (The illustrations associated with the color coding in this system are inappropriate and should be disregarded.)

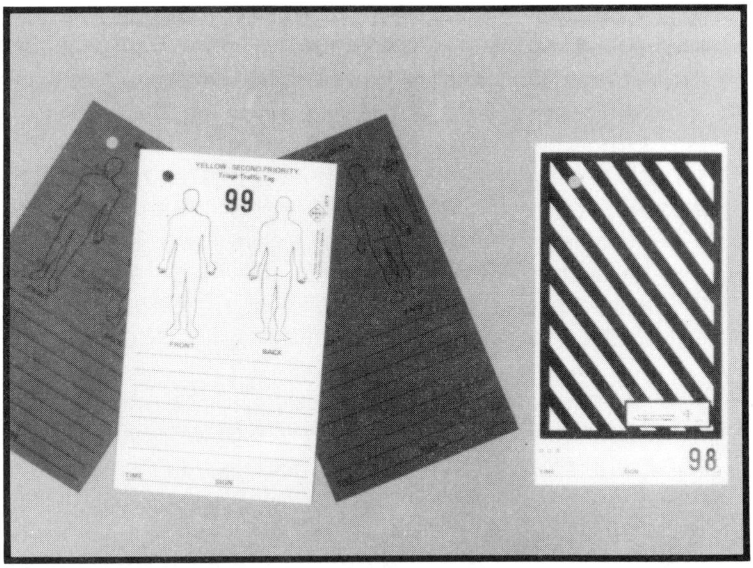

The second system has separate tags for each priority. Only one tag is placed on the patient. If a patient deteriorates, a second tag is added and responders react to the higher priority color.

The third system is a combination of the first two. It uses a stapled package of individual tags. The responder tears off the appropriate color and places it on the patient. The remaining colored cards in the pack are discarded. Instead of a black tag, a grey one is included for dead patients.

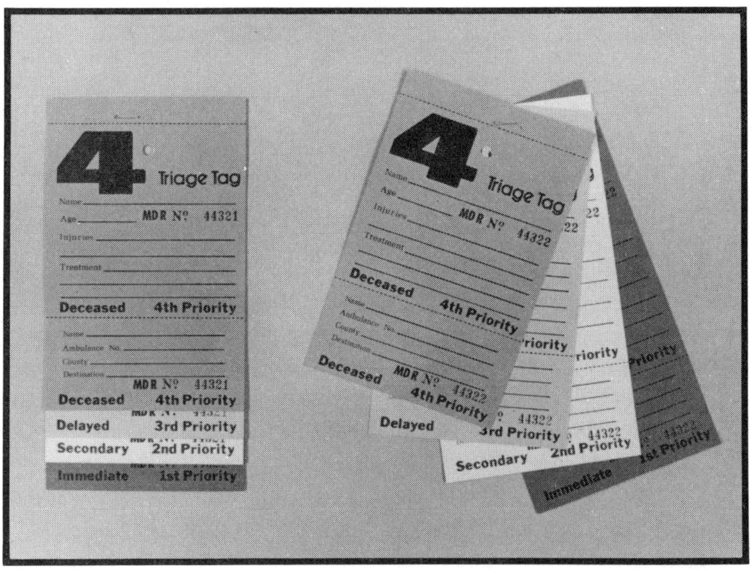

None of these systems is entirely satisfactory. None, for example, provides for any indication that a primary survival scan has been performed. In a closed incident this usually does not present a problem because responders move from row to row. In an open or complex incident, however, it does. At one drill we witnessed 8 different responders do a primary scan on a single patient, since there was no way of knowing who had been examined and who had not. We now use a second tag, a simple kraft mailing tag available at any stationery store, to indicate that such a scan has been done. Since another problem with existing triage tags is lack of adequate space for assessment information, this second tag may also be used to record such data.

Unfortunately, the pack and tear-off systems do not provide for *downgrading* a patient's priority—e.g., a Red who, on more careful assessment, proves to be Yellow. Should this occur, a new pack or tear-off tag must be obtained.

An additional problem with both the pack and the tear-off tag results from the use of a patient numbering system in the tens or hundreds of thousands. Most people cannot easily remember numbers of this magnitude. Numbers in the single tag system run from 1 to 100. Unfortunately, however, this sequence is repeated in each color, allowing for confusion.

Some tags provide space for hospital treatment information. This demonstrates a misunderstanding of their purpose. Triage tags are for field triage and field information. Hospital personnel should disregard field triage priorities since they are outdated by the time the patient arrives.

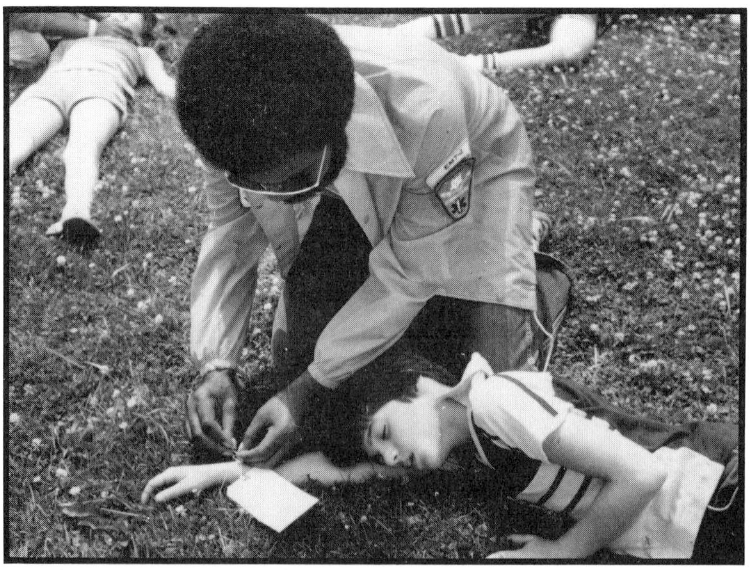

The stapled, layered tag packs have criteria for urgency printed on the back. This is both space-consuming and misleading. For example, cardiac arrest is indicated as a "first priority" Red condition. Anyone familiar with mass casualty triage knows that a patient in cardiac arrest is considered dead and should not be given treatment.

Basic triage, or the sorting of patients into color-coded priority categories, is done against a set of "absolute" definitions. It is *not* based upon "relative" considerations, i.e., relative to other patients. A patient *is* or *is not* urgent, regardless of the condition or number of other patients. A second reason that basic triage is done this way is the structure of the situation. As patients arrive at the collecting station, each must be rapidly categorized. One cannot wait until 15 to 20 patients have arrived in order to place them in a sequence of relative priority, nor could one retain the pertinent information. Instead, as they arrive, patients are categorized into groups of urgency against the preconceived standard. Then, from the more manageable numbers within each group, the Triage Officer can make "relative" decisions, e.g., which 2 Red category patients should be transported next.

Nothing should interfere with the independence of each decision. For instance, any misgivings that there are *too many Reds* must *not* translate into a change in classification criteria. It must be understood that the number of patients in each category is based solely on the nature of their injuries.

The major factor determining the quality of triage is how well the definitions of each color-coded priority group are applied. This appears to have a greater effect on salvage rate than differences in skill. Therefore, it is key that the reader study the following criteria and understand them.

Red Category—First Priority, Most Urgent

Patients should be classified as Red priority if they meet *3* criteria. First, the injuries are such that life-threatening shock and/or hypoxia is present or imminent. Second, the patient can be stabilized without the need for constant or labor-intensive care. And third, the patient has a high probability of survival if given immediate care and rapidly transported. Patients that do not meet all 3 of these criteria should not be classified as Red. It is important to note that patients with catastrophic injuries of the head or chest do not meet these criteria. They have a poor chance of survival and usually need constant intensive care. They should, therefore, *not be placed in the Red category*.

A good example of a Red category patient is the following:

A teenage boy has a piece of wood impaled in his abdomen.

skin: pale, cool, moist
breathing quality: shallow, slow, guarded
pulse quality: rapid, thready, regular
neurological status: well oriented; feels pain; pupils equal and reactive (E/R)
medical history: not applicable
further examination: not applicable

This patient quite obviously meets the Red category criteria. He is certainly urgent and presents a clinical picture of shock. One must assume that he still has intra-abdominal bleeding, but is not yet in shock deep enough to alter his state of consciousness materially. If, however, he is not treated rapidly, he could easily decline into irreversible shock and die. If treated rapidly, either surgically or by removal of the wooden object and the use of anti-shock trousers, his survival is almost assured—based upon his age and injury.

Yellow Category—Second Priority, Urgent

The Yellow category will be transported after the Red. Two different types of patients are placed in the Yellow category. One type is called *Yellow* and the other, *Yellow Prime*. Both types have equal second-priority urgency.

Yellow category patients are: first, patients whose injuries have systemic implications and effects, but who are not *yet* in life-threatening shock or hypoxia. Unless countered, however, systemic decline will ensue. Second, they are patients who appear able to withstand a 45- to 60-minute wait in the field without immediate life risk.

A good example of a Yellow category patient is the following:

A female, 25, has multiple fractures of both lower legs. Fractures are closed. She is sitting up on the ground.

skin: pale, dry, warm
breathing quality: slightly faster than normal, good air exchange
pulse quality: full, regular, slightly rapid
neurological status: pupils E/R; well oriented; unaltered state of consciousness; moves and speaks spontaneously
medical history: not applicable
further examination: no other abnormal findings, no other injuries

Although some shock is present, this patient is compensating well and appears to be able to withstand 45 to 60 minutes of waiting (particularly if given support treatment for shock). The extent of the fractures makes her urgent enough to be a second priority since the shock could deepen, causing further deterioration (and transfer to Red).

It is important to note that sometimes the distinctions between a Red and Yellow category patient are subtle. This patient's level of consciousness, her sitting position, and her warm, dry skin are the basis for the assumption that she can afford to wait. All Yellow patients should be rechecked periodically. Patients who progress into more advanced shock should be reclassified as Red.

Yellow Prime patients are the catastrophically injured. They are placed in this second priority on a totally different basis. Many of these patients are among the most urgent. However, based upon their very poor chance for survival regardless of care, they are relegated to the second priority and are not transported until after the highly salvageable Red patients. Emotionally, this is the most difficult consideration associated with Mass Casualty Incidents, but its overall effect is to increase the number of survivors.

A good example of a Yellow Prime patient would be the following victim:

A male, 65, has massive intrathoracic injury. Major skull fractures are apparent.

skin:	cyanotic, cold and moist; appears translucent
breathing quality:	rapid, shallow, and irregular
pulse quality:	radial pulses are absent; carotid pulses are palpable, rapid, and weak
neurological status:	patient is unconscious; does not react to stimuli
medical history:	not available
further examination:	reveals multiple fractures of the lower legs, silverfork fracture of the left wrist, and flail chest

There is no question that this patient is in deep shock and has various catastrophic injuries. The type and extent of injury, coupled with his age, give him a very poor chance of survival (even if he were the only victim). His needs require a great deal of labor-intensive care and will tie up many field and hospital workers.

It is important to remember that *Yellow category patients are not abandoned or left as if non-urgent*. They *are* urgent and are transported on a priority basis *immediately after Red*—the more salvageable urgent group. Some international military triage systems categorize the catastrophically injured with the dead. In normal MCIs this is inappropriate. These patients should receive care and transportation ahead of patients with no urgent need.

Yellow and Yellow Prime patients should be placed in separate rows in the Yellow area. This will aid in identifying each for care and retriage when additional medical help is available. It also facilitates transportation. One Yellow and one Yellow Prime patient are usually transported together. Transporting 2 Yellow Primes at the same time will cause patient-management problems en route.

Green Category—Third Priority, Non-Urgent

These are patients with localized injuries that do not commonly have an immediate systemic implication. Experience shows that if these patients are given a minimum of care they generally do not deteriorate. Generally, this type of patient can wait up to several hours to receive care—without danger to life or limb. Patients who would fit this definition after a minimum of care (such as splinting and immobilization of a limb), should also be included. One must remember that in a very short period these patients will receive some aid and attention (although of a limited nature) in the field. They will, however, endure substantial delays prior to transport to a hospital—either because they will not be moved until after all patients with any degree of urgency, or because they will be transported to a distant, outlying hospital (bypassing the near facilities). The term "walking wounded," sometimes applied to Green category patients, is both unprofessional and misleading. Whether a patient is or is not ambulatory should not be a consideration for urgency—only for how they will move or be moved. A patient who presents a clinical picture of shock due to multiple fractures of the upper extremities and no injuries to the lower extremities should be a Yellow or Red category patient. Conversely, a patient who has sustained only a simple fracture of the lower leg and has no progressive shock or deteriorating condition, should be placed in the Green category even though he is not ambulatory.

A good example of a Green category patient is the following:

A young woman in her mid-twenties is walking around. She cannot move her right arm and has pain at her shoulder.

skin: color good; warm, dry
breathing quality: rapid, regular; normal depth
pulse quality: rapid, full, regular at both radials
neurological status: well oriented; pupils E/R
medical history: not applicable
further examination: indicates point tenderness upon palpation of the right clavicle

This young woman appears to have a possible fracture of the right clavicle without any other injury. By the proper application of either a modified under-the-arm sling and swathe or a posterior figure-eight bandage of the shoulder, the arm and shoulder can be supported and immobilized. Once this is done, no deterioration or progessive shock is expected, and with a minimum of care she can sustain several hours of waiting for definitive treatment without risk to life or limb. Note that she has full, regular, normal palpable pulses at *both* radials. Specifically, she has unimpaired circulation distal to the injury site.

Black Category—Dead, Non-Urgent

The Black category represents victims who are dead. In an MCI, any unresponsive patient who has no spontaneous circulation is classified as dead without further resuscitative efforts. No distinction between clinical and biological death can be made. The delivery of CPR simply cannot be afforded. (A possible exception would be a patient under 45 years of age, who is witnessed or still viable and who is in arrest secondary to hemorrhagic shock. The application of anti-shock trousers may produce enough venous return to resuscitate him and reinstate spontaneous circulation. Should this patient then respond, he would be classified as Red.)

Dead victims should *not* be placed at the collecting station near the injured. A location at a reasonable distance should be designated as a morgue.

Other Factors Affecting Triage

Besides the *nature* and *urgency* (based upon the present systemic condition), the prognosis—and therefore, the categorization—must include some other factors relative to the patient's overall condition. Triage must also be sensitive to considerations of the victim's appearance and his general state of health. In healthy people, certain injuries have a good prognosis. However, the same injury in a person with poor health may not have a high survival expectation. If the Triage Officer is sophisticated in his skills, the patient's age, general health, and physical condition will all be factored in. Rather than making complex distinctions based on age, it is more appropriate to use 4 groupings:

1. Under 15 years of age
2. From 16 to 45 years of age
3. From 46 to 65 years of age
4. Over 65 years of age

Field triage is also affected by the intervention levels available at the site. Both the qualifications of the individuals and the availability of key supplies and equipment (such as IVs and anti-shock trousers) will affect categorization.

Anti-shock trousers serve as a good example. If they are *not* available, an otherwise healthy 20-year-old victim with only intra-abdominal blunt injury associated with a clinical picture of shock and a falling systolic pressure under 90 mm Hg is a top priority Red category patient. If he is rapidly taken to a hospital and placed in anti-shock trousers, he will in all probability survive. If he is left in the field for a sustained period he will probably deteriorate until irreversible shock occurs. If, on the other hand, the same patient has anti-shock trousers applied in the field, restoring his systolic pressure to 100 to 110 mm Hg with an associated improvement in his presenting clinical picture (and if his condition remains stable), he can safely be held in the field with proper monitoring until more-urgent patients are transported.

Reviewing Triage Categories

The triage categories and the underlying principles for the categorization can be reviewed using a simple "branching" chart.

The first criteria is urgency. Is the patient urgent?

URGENT

NO **YES**

Victims are categorized *not* urgent either because their injury is local and not commonly associated with deterioration, or because they are dead. All victims whose injuries have systemic physiological implications *are* urgent. Therefore, patients who are not urgent are either in the Green or the Black category, and patients who are urgent are either in the Red or Yellow category.

URGENT

NO	**YES**
Green or *Black*	*Red* or *Yellow*

The distinction between non-urgent living patients and dead patients is quite apparent and needs no further discussion. The distinction between Red—most urgent, and Yellow—urgent but second priority, is complex. In application, this distinction is often sensitive to individual judgment and diagnosis, and to general clinical impressions. The concepts, however, are easily separable.

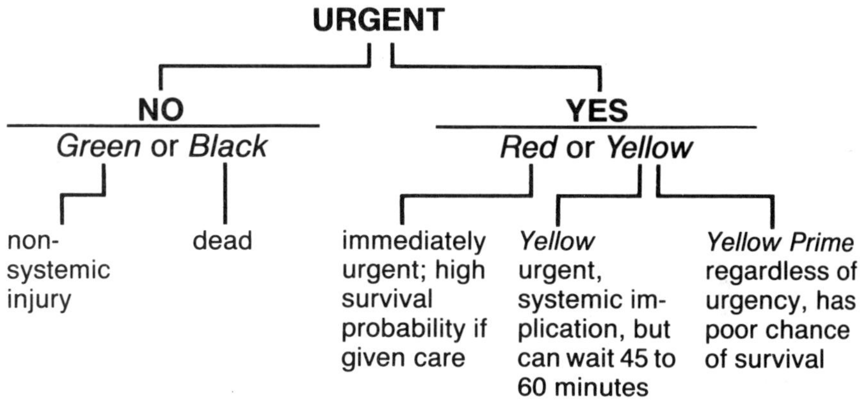

It is important to remember that once a patient has been classified by category he should be tagged and placed in an area or row of patients of that category. The orderly segregation of patients by priority is a necessary part of triage. Random location of tagged patients makes the identifying of priority patients next to impossible. Where patients are not physically placed in rows by category, triage does not work effectively.

Reviewing the Triage Sequence

First, all patients are given a rapid primary survival scan. This really constitutes one type of partial triage and includes treatment to stop bleeding, open airways, and/or position patients to avoid airway impairment from fluids.

A second kind of sorting deals with how patients "come out"—how they are extricated or are selected from where they lie. In a bus, plane, fire, or building collapse, patients will often come out on the basis of considerations unrelated to medical triage. For example, generally the first few victims taken off a bus are moved because they are in the way and impede the egress of others.

Then, as patients arrive at the collecting station, they are tagged and placed in rows. This is done fairly rapidly and without careful, in-depth examination by the Triage Officer.

Triage is an ongoing process that must include the constant revision of categories based upon either patient change (most commonly deterioration) or upon reconsideration based on more careful examination (as time allows). Therefore, after patients are in the rows, quite a number of them will be reclassified by the EMTs or physicians in the collecting area. These recommended reclassifications should be addressed to the Triage Officer and, if agreed to, should result in the retagging and moving of the patient.

At this point, the Triage Officer will be dealing with one category at a time: first Red, then Yellow. Now the considerations within this smaller subgroup of victims become relative. As each ambulance becomes available, for example, the Triage Officer decides which 2 Red patients are the most urgent and therefore, should be the next to go. This process, plus the previously mentioned reclassification based upon further examination, remediates any errors caused by the arbitrary judgments required during rapid absolute triage. This earlier step, however, is necessitated by the sudden patient influxes that occur at the collecting station and by the need to establish the subgrouping. It provides the order and structure necessary to allow for meaningful relative triage considerations. Experience shows when these 2 steps—rapid absolute triage followed by more careful relative triage from each row—are not performed, triage falls apart. If only the rapid triage is done, mis-sequencing occurs. When the first triage is done too slowly, "haul and run" transportation of untriaged patients results. Either of these errors produces the same result: increased morbidity and mortality.

Remember that the categories are only subsets in a continuum. In essence, they are one continuous ordering. The first Yellow patient comes immediately after the last Red, and the first Green immediately follows the last Yellow.

A good general rule when in doubt about a borderline decision (e.g., determining whether a patient is Yellow or Red) is not to delay or ponder. Instead, *quickly elect the more urgent of the two*. The worst errors always come from doing the task too slowly or too timidly. The Triage Officer must be experienced in rapid field assessment and in making rapid field decisions, and must have secure EMS leadership skills.

In some cases, essentially nonmedical considerations must also be factored into the priority assigned a given patient. Should a uniformed responder become seriously injured, or for example, develop substernal pain, that responder should be considered a Red and be one of the next patients transported. Similarly, if a close relative of a responder is one of the urgent victims, the relative should be designated Red and be transported promptly. Even though these patients may, upon medical considerations, not war-

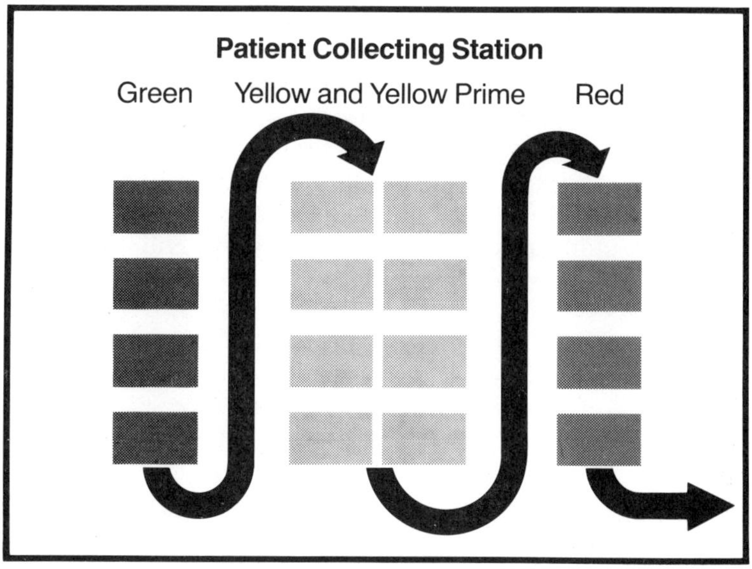

rant such a high priority, they should be transported to minimize the anxiety, subsequent distraction, and possible inefficiency of responders in the field. A responder with a close relative or fellow responder injured in the field represents a potential threat to calm, orderly operations at the site. For the same reasons, a hysterical patient, or a patient accompanied by a hysterical relative, should be given a higher priority than his medical condition might warrant.

It is also wise, because of the emotional factors involved when children are injured, to transport a child before an adult *in the same triage classification*. This policy has a positive effect on responder's morale.

It should be clear that field triage categorization is a system limited solely to establishing priorities in the field and for transportation from the field. At the hospital, patients should be totally retriaged. Significant time has elapsed since *field triage* occurred. The patient has been jostled and moved. Much more accurate diagnosis is possible based upon a better environment, fewer patients to deal with, more extensive diagnostic tools, and much more advanced medical skills. Considerations of hospital triage are discussed in Chapter 11, *Hospital Disaster Plans*.

Practicing Triage Decisions

It is important that *all* EMS personnel be trained in mass casualty triage. Only if each EMT understands the triage goals will he be able to perform his individual role efficiently.

Mass casualty triage cannot be learned passively, since the task includes relating the generalities to specific patient conditions and injuries. It is a practical skill—like splinting or bandaging—that must be applied and practiced. On the ensuing pages, you will find sample patient descriptions taken from *Triage Practice Cards*. Read each and determine in which category you would classify each patient. You should be able to explain why you selected a particular category.

TRIAGE PRACTICE **PATIENT DESCRIPTION #1**

A young man states he cannot feel or move his legs.

skin: pale, cool, moist
breathing quality: slow, normal depth, regular
pulse quality: rapid, full, regular
neurological status: well oriented; pupils E/R; hand grip equal and strong
medical history: not applicable
further examination: no reaction to painful stimuli in legs

TRIAGE PRACTICE **PATIENT DESCRIPTION #2**

A woman in her twenties has had her left leg partially amputated.

skin: cyanotic, cool, moist
breathing quality: shallow, regular; rate not alarming
pulse quality: very rapid, weak, regular
neurological status: drifts in and out; responds to verbal stimuli only occasionally
medical history: not available
further examination: hemorrhage has been extensive

TRIAGE PRACTICE **PATIENT DESCRIPTION #3**

A man has a steel rod about 2 feet long impaled in his thigh.

skin: pale, dry, cool
breathing quality: rapid, deep, regular
pulse quality: rapid, full, regular
neurological status: well oriented; feels pain; pupils E/R
medical history: not applicable
further examination: minor bleeding from wound; no palpable fracture

TRIAGE PRACTICE **PATIENT DESCRIPTION #4**

A boy cannot extend his leg due to severe pain in the knee.

skin: pale, dry, cool
breathing quality: rapid, deep, regular
pulse quality: bounding, regular
neurological status: well oriented; feels pain; pupils E/R
medical history: not applicable
further examination: pulses distal to knee full and regular

TRIAGE PRACTICE **PATIENT DESCRIPTION #5**

A woman in her thirties is unconscious and has severe facial lacerations, and appears to have suffered chest injuries.

skin: cyanotic, cool, moist
breathing quality: absent
pulse quality: absent
neurological status: unresponsive; pupils are fixed and dilated
medical history: not available
further examination: patient is unresponsive

TRIAGE PRACTICE **PATIENT DESCRIPTION #6**

An elderly woman is walking around supporting her right wrist.

skin: normal color; cool, dry
breathing quality: rapid, deep, regular
pulse quality: rapid, full, regular
neurological status: well oriented; feels pain; pupils E/R
medical history: not applicable
further examination: "silver fork" appearance of right wrist

TRIAGE PRACTICE **PATIENT DESCRIPTION #7**

A 35-year-old woman has had a tourniquet applied to her right arm to control hemorrhage due to multiple lacerations.

skin: cool, moist, clammy
breathing quality: rapid, full, regular
pulse quality: rapid, weak, irregular
neurological status: disoriented; reponds to verbal stimuli; responds to pain
medical history: not applicable
further examination: BP 76/54

TRIAGE PRACTICE **PATIENT DESCRIPTION #8**

A middle-aged man has suffered severe chest trauma.

skin: cool, moist, cyanotic
breathing quality: rapid, shallow, irregular
pulse quality: regular, rapid, weak
neurological status: disoriented; pupils equal and react slowly; feels pain; responds to verbal stimuli
medical history: not available
further examination: paradoxical motion of chest; BP 70/40

TRIAGE PRACTICE **PATIENT DESCRIPTION #9**

A teenage girl is applying direct pressure to a wound and elevating her right arm to control the hemorrhage. Her clothes are covered with blood.

skin: cool, pale, dry
breathing quality: rapid, deep, regular
pulse quality: full, regular, rapid
neurological status: well oriented; pupils E/R
medical history: not applicable
further examination: BP 100/68

TRIAGE PRACTICE **PATIENT DESCRIPTION #10**

A teenage girl is crying out in pain. Her left leg is severely angulated between the knee and ankle.

skin: color good; dry, warm
breathing quality: normal depth, slightly rapid, regular
pulse quality: rapid, full, regular
neurological status: pupils E/R; feels pain; well oriented
medical history: penicillin allergy
further examination: skin warm distal to fracture; distal pulse full and regular

Triage is very much like playing chess. The more one does it, the more skilled and sophisticated one becomes. Additional factors and possibilities become apparent and dimensions of skill and fine judgment not previously perceived become apparent. One never seems to learn enough about it.

An excellent way to develop skills is with the use of *Triage Practice Cards* similar to the preceeding patient descriptions. Working in a small group, each person takes 3 or 4 cards. One by one, each person reads a card and explains why he or she would put the patient in a given category. The other members of the group agree or disagree and explain why. Ensuing discussions, defending or challenging each choice, represent a valuable triage learning experience.

Chapter 7

SKILLS IN RAPID FIELD ASSESSMENT

Daily and MCI Assessment

Normal patient assessment methods must be modified in a Mass Casualty Incident. Daily prehospital patient assessment develops a detailed picture and history in a sequence based upon potential urgency. It is performed primarily by one responder, at one time and in one place, following an extensive checklist. Although normal assessment is done rapidly, detailed measurements and a relatively complete examination are involved in assessing multitrauma victims.

In a Mass Casualty Incident time is of the essence, both as it relates to the patient being assessed and as it relates to other patients awaiting the responder's attention. Patient assessment is the basis for triage, but the converse is also true: the process of triage provides the basis for the level of the assessment done at any point.

In a Mass Casualty Incident assessment is segmented into different levels, to be done at different times. This assures that *all* patients will be checked to one level of urgency before *any* are checked in more detail. Furthermore, it involves moving to more intensive levels of examination with all urgent patients before doing the same with apparently stable, non-urgent patients. This distributes the limited available personnel in the most effective way and increases the number of patients stabilized. It also reduces the time from insult to stabilization.

The mass casualty examination is also characterized by a more rapid method, which should not be misconstrued as being less careful or accurate. Instead, as in all urgent, multiple-trauma cases, the assessment is reduced to key measurements. The resulting information is more meaningful than a mass of detail that is not germane to whatever is the most serious or threatening condition. The measurement of blood pressure serves as a good example. Whether a patient has a BP of 120/80, 130/86, or 110/77 does not tell us much. More important are broader questions:

1. Does the patient have spontaneous circulation and blood pressure in an acceptable range?
2. Is the systolic pressure over 100 mm Hg? Is it over 70 to 80 mm Hg? Or is the patient in progressive shock? Is the shock so severe that vital organ hypoperfusion must be assumed?

In only a few patients—and only when other, more rapidly discernable signs so direct—might one quickly need to know the exact systolic and diastolic pressures (i.e., patients who appear to be in marked hypertension, have suspected brain damage, have fluid overload, or who may be suspected of having a cardiac tamponade).

Rather than the more conservative daily practice of checking an essentially constant list of items, one checks a more abbreviated list on all patients and examines further only what appears relevant. Consider next ventilatory and circulatory quality, which must be checked on all patients. During an MCI, additional examination occurs only if it appears that the findings may relate to deterioration in ventilation, circulation, neurological function, or biochemical balance. The mass casualty assessment is stripped down to what one really needs to know—namely, indexes of potential life threat. It focuses on evaluating the condition and level of vital functions by examining the patient to find out where he is in the progression from health to death; checking for the patient's ability to provide for his own vital needs; identifying any pathophysiology that threatens or compromises maintenance of life needs; and correcting or compensating for any loss or impairment.

It is important to emphasize that mass casualty assessment is directed at *locating conditions that cause patients to die*. Rather than completely documenting each and every injury or problem, it seeks to find what the patient's stabilization needs are. The immobilization on boards of all seriously injured patients and all patients with an altered state of consciousness makes the location of each possible fracture a waste of time—time that is urgently needed for the care of other patients.

Two harsh facts of life about an MCI must be understood. First, due to constraints of time and available personnel, one must deal with *probabilities* and make certain assumptions that have historically proven to be true. This kind of statistical "numbers game" always presents some danger to the individual exception. However, time doesn't allow one to act otherwise, both for the individual patient and the others urgently in need of care. (Note: This practice is not entirely alien to daily emergency care. For example, when faced with a patient in cardiac arrest that has prevailed for several minutes, metabolic respiratory acidosis must be assumed. Urgency then dictates sodium bicarbonate as part of the accepted course of initial treatment *prior to laboratory results*.)

Second, our diagnostic methods must be more rapid and must focus on what it is vital to discover. Again, blood pressure will serve as a good example. The palpation of a radial pulse (and, in the absence thereof, the femoral and/or carotid pulses) will tell us if there is spontaneous circulation, tachycardia, normocardia, or bradycardia. Presence of a palpable radial pulse indicates a systolic blood pressure of over 80 mm Hg. Presence of a palpable carotid pulse indicates a systolic blood pressure that is over 60 mm Hg.

Similarly, the use of the capillary refill test will give us a quick, reliable impression of whether or not the patient is hypovolemic.

Segmented Assessment Procedure

In an MCI, patient field assessment is broken into 3 parts.

1. The primary survival scan
2. The rapid triage assessment
3. The more thorough assessment at the collecting station

For a given patient, each of these parts occurs at a different time and at a different location, and involves a different EMT. After these steps, all patients are monitored for signs of change. In cases where personnel with skills more advanced than those of the responders making the original assessment become available in the field, a fourth, "advanced," assessment may occur.

Each of these 3 parts has a different main objective.

PRIMARY SURVIVAL SCAN*

The major objective is to assess all patients rapidly. This means identifying and remediating any major hemorrhage, airway obstruction, or other ventilatory problem that can be dealt with instantly—e.g., hemorrhage that can be controlled by direct pressure; airway obstruction that can be rectified by repositioning (moving the head out of flexure and/or placing the patient into a coma position); ventilatory threat that can be handled by clearing the mouth and nose or removing objects from a victim's chest.

*The term *primary survival scan* is unique to this text. It would be misleading to use a term of the art such as *primary survey*.

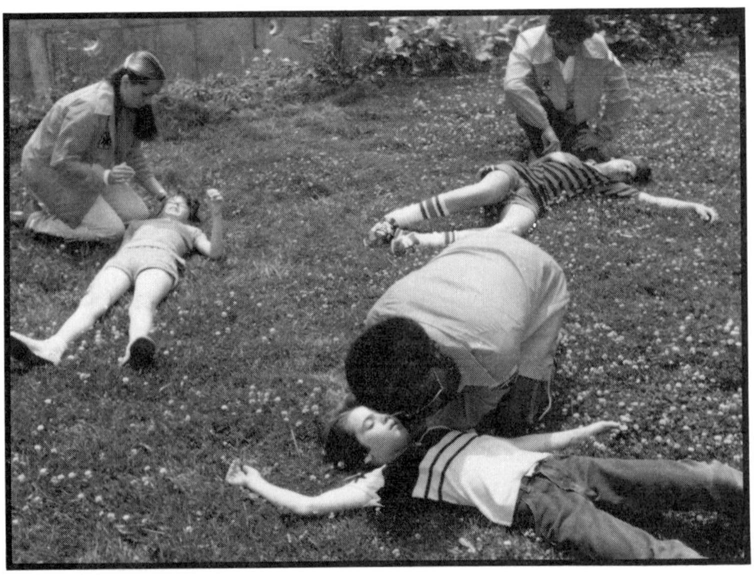

RAPID TRIAGE ASSESSMENT

Once all patients have been scanned, the next assessment step can be implemented. How this is done will vary depending on whether the incident is *open* or *closed* and upon environmental factors. In a closed incident, patients are handled in an order determined by their location in the wreckage and their ease of removal. In an open situation an attempt is made to locate and transport more urgent patients to the collecting station first.

This assessment step has the following major purposes:

- Separate the urgent patients from the non-urgent patients (urgent: *yes/no*).
- Rapidly triage the urgent patients into categories of urgency (Yellow, Yellow Prime, or Red).
- Locate, on a need-to-know basis, key injuries to determine how to move patients onto rigid boards (C-spine: *yes/no*).

This assessment is limited to the immediate interim need to move and categorize patients rapidly, thereby arriving at a realistic number to deal with at a time. Remember, errors will be corrected later as a thorough assessment is made.

To speed this assessment 3 prime indexes are used:

- Injuries that can be found rapidly
- Clinical impressions of level of shock and ventilation
- Symptoms or conditions that generally have poor salvage rates

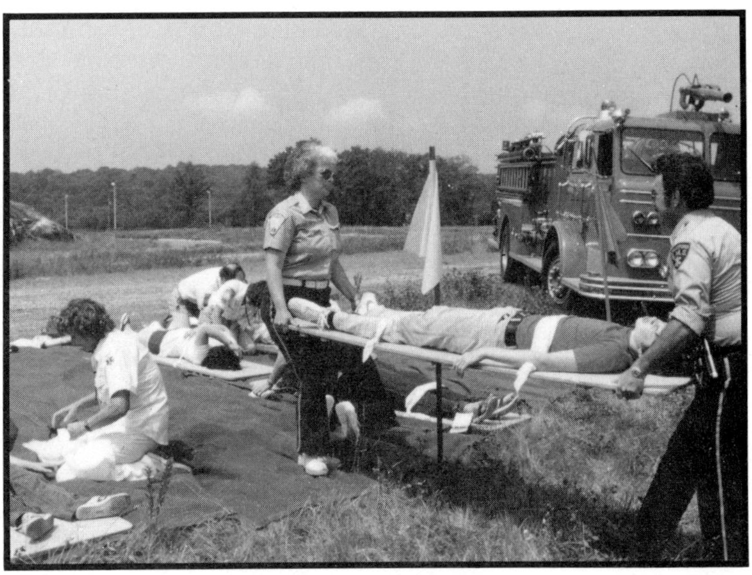

The separation of urgent from non-urgent can be done by the experienced EMT in under a minute. This is based upon:

- the overt injuries;
- visible vital function indicators;
- use of pulse to determine whether the patient has tachycardia or bradycardia;
- whether the systolic BP is more than 60, 70, or 80 mm Hg;
- the depth and rate of respiration, coupled with a rapid evaluation of airway and breathing quality; and
- a combination of the AVPU system (to evaluate level of consciousness) and the clinical impression (from skin and lip color, lucidity, etc.) to determine at what point between normality and deep shock the patient appears to be.

The consideration of immobilization (C-spine: *yes/no*) has to be made on the basis of apparent injury and/or mechanism of injury.

Distinctions among the urgent are more judgmental and more difficult to make. The examiner must determine which of the following 3 definitions *best* describes the patient.

- Very urgent and very salvageable (Red)
- Urgent, salvageable, and can wait 45 minutes (Yellow)
- Urgent or very urgent, poor probability of salvage (Yellow Prime)

Conditions Associated with Poor Salvage

Rapidly identifying those patients who, regardless of care, have poor salvageability is difficult both emotional and intellectually. The following list provides a guideline to apparent conditions that are known to have a very poor salvage rate.

1. Severe open fracture of the cranium (with exposed brain tissue)
2. Gross deformity of the head (i.e., loss of ovoid shape)
3. Increased intracranial pressure (i.e., patients displaying blown, pupil and/or rising blood pressure with slowing pulse rate)
4. Cervical fracture with quadriplegia (may be Yellow or Yellow Prime, depending on other injuries)
5. Any loss of maintenance of airway that cannot be cleared by the Heimlich maneuver, rapid suctioning, insertion of an airway, or positioning
6. Substantial burns of face associated with inhalation of superheated air or other hot gases

7. Any crushing injury to the trachea associated with dyspnea and cyanosis
8. Any catastrophic injury of the chest—anterior or posterior
9. Any *substantial* breach of the thoracic cavity
10. Any advanced pulmonary edema/CHF
11. Massive generalized subcutaneous emphysema
12. Any cardiogenic shock
13. Cardiac tamponade
14. Sucking wounds of the abdomen (breached diaphragm)
15. Severe evisceration with spillage of intestinal contents
16. Catastrophic multiple injury to the trunk
17. Substantial multiple injury to any patient in poor general health, or to one with significant systemic disease.

MORE THOROUGH ASSESSMENT AT THE COLLECTING STATION

The third "assessment" represents the first examination that is close to normal daily EMS patient assessment. Although the assessment is thorough, its methodology has been abridged so that it is less time consuming. Remember, the patient is already on a rigid board—that is, he has been reduced to a normal anatomical position and is supported and immobilized. Therefore, individual fractures of the arms and legs, with the exception of the knee and femur, have been stabilized. Similarly, the 2 earlier asssessments have already dealt with airway, spontaneous ventilation, control of

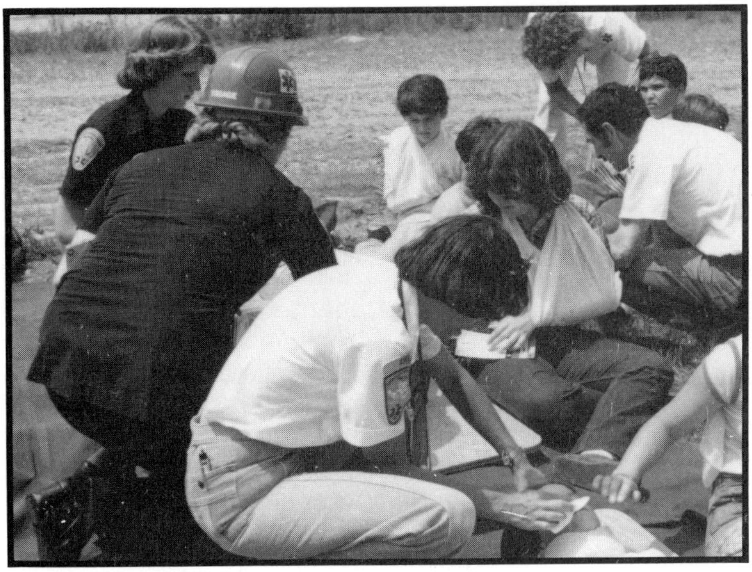

major external bleeding, and C-spine immobilization, as indicated. With all of the above understood, in most cases a rapid, multi-trauma assessment will be made. The remaining fears are airway/ventilatory compromise, internal hemorrhage, and progressive shock.

1. Look at the patient and get an instant impression from his appearance. Does he move spontaneously? Is he conscious? Is he in shock? Ask the patient where he hurts or is injured. Note major obvious injuries. What condition or conclusions caused this patient to be placed in the color category?

2. If the patient is unresponsive, quickly recheck the airway. Check for spontaneous ventilation. Evaluate chest rise and estimate if the rate is adequate (over 10 to 12 per minute). Observe if collateral muscles are used in ventilation. Is there apparent air hunger, dyspnea, fulminating pulmonary edema, gurgling, etc.?

Simultaneously, auscultate the upper lung fields, left and right, for adequacy of air exchange. Examine the mucosa of mouth and lips for color (cyanosis?) and moisture.

3. Palpate the radial pulse to estimate systolic BP. (If not present, palpate the carotid.) Gain an impression of pulse quality and estimate if the rate is indicative of tachycardia, normocardia, or bradycardia.

4. Note skin color and temperature; perform a capillary refill test to ascertain if the patient appears normovolemic or hypovolemic. Observe neck veins, relative to patient's postural position.

5. Bare and examine the chest. Auscultate the lungs for normal breath sounds, normal resonance, and for quality of respiration (rhonchi? rales?), etc. Palpate above the clavicles and neck for the presence of subcutaneous emphysema; ascertain that the trachea is in the midline position; examine the chest for proper motion and for signs of injury. Palpate the sternum and ribs. You are essentially examining for loss of continuity of the thoracic cavity or chest wall; and to determine if the patient has a flail chest, any signs of paradoxical movement, a pneumothorax, hemopneumothorax, or a tension pneumothorax.

Converse with the patient throughout this examination. His responses will provide an indication of his level of consciousness as he provides a history of the incident.

6. Evaluate neurological status and complete AVPU.

A—Alert: speaks and moves spontaneously (Already observed.)
V—Responds to verbal stimulus (Already observed.)
P—Responds to painful stimulus (Check if patient does not move limb in response to verbal stimulus.)
U—Unresponsive (Already observed.)

Check pupils—size and reactiveness.

If indicated: take a more accurate BP, count pulse, etc.; provide needed systemic treatment; start IVs, apply MAST, give oxygen, seal open pneumothorax, etc.

7. Examine head, neck, face, mouth, and ears.
8. Examine abdomen and pelvis.
9. Examine extremities *for circulation*.
10. Where indicated, check extremities for response. If the earlier neurological exam (AVPU) showed an altered state of consciousness, check for the best response of eyes, verbal, and motor.
11. Obtain succinct, pertinent history.

A—Allergies (to medicines only)
M—Medications currently taken
P—Past key conditions/illness
L—Last meal? What?
E—Pertinent events preceeding and during the incident

It is key to note that constant monitoring and re-evaluation should occur at the patient collecting station.

The above abridged assessment, when performed by a skilled EMT, takes no more than 2 to 3 minutes.

A patient who shows any real urgency should *not* be held in order to complete the assessment. Only hold patients at the field sorting station to furnish key intervention, *or* because others must be transported first. The more rapidly patients who cannot be stabilized in the field are moved to a near hospital, the better their chance of survival.

Chapter 8

SKILLS FOR RAPID PACKAGING

Stabilizing Multitrauma Patients

As a rule, a majority of the patients in a Mass Casualty Incident will be multiple-trauma victims. When a building collapses, when 2 trains collide, when a bomb goes off, most of the people who are caught in the resulting destruction must inevitably be injured in several places. If ignition is also a factor, the patients may have injuries from burns and/or from inhalation of superheated air, smoke, gases, and toxic fumes.

By definition, a Mass Casualty Incident precludes time-consuming treatment of injuries before the patients are moved. It is impossible to care properly for victims where they lie. Field efforts must be directed to triage—sorting and moving the patients several times in an effort to get them to hospitals in order of established priorities. This means that all patients must be stabilized and packaged for transport quickly, efficiently, and effectively. Since patients must be moved prior to assessment, a pessimistic approach is essential: assume that anyone not categorized Green is multiply injured.

When faced with a large number of patients, most of whom are suspected multiple-trauma victims, it is impossible to locate and stabilize each broken bone for every patient. All attention at this stage must go toward locating and stabilizing life-threatening systemic problems involving ventilation, circulation, and shock. Broken bones should be dealt with only if they threaten ventilation, systemic circulation, or circulation to a limb. In an MCI, all other broken bones are considered nonpriority injuries. The treatment can wait—so long as the breaks are immobilized.

In order to immobilize every possible broken bone without unnecessary delay, fasten every suspected multiple-trauma patient to a long board.

Use of Long Boards

1. As has already been suggested, a long board will immobilize and support every part of a patient's body, thus preventing further damage to broken bones and surrounding tissues.

2. Use of long boards will also simplify moving the patient from place to place. It has been calculated that a victim of an MCI may be moved upwards of 10 times: from the immediate scene of the disaster to a triage area; from one row to another of the triage area as he is reclassified, possibly several times; onto the ambulance cot; into and out of the ambulance; into the hospital triage center; to the Emergency Room; to X-ray; to a treatment room; to the OR, etc. By keeping a patient on "his" board until definitive treatment at

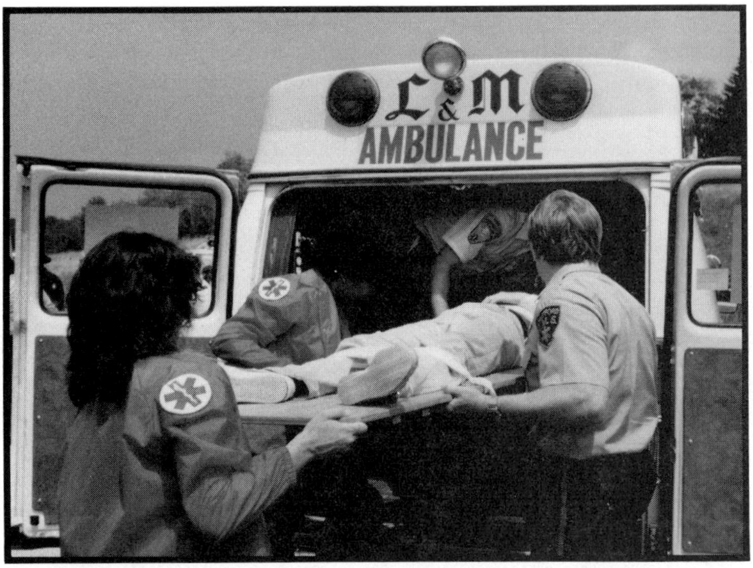

the hospital is underway or has been completed, we minimize risk of damage *and* facilitate efficient movement. Folding canvas litters do not make acceptable substitutes for boards for the following reasons:

a. They are too flexible, and permit excessive movement of the body.
b. The canvas weakens with age, and may rip.

Ambulance cots, which are also too flexible, are not acceptable substitutes for boards either. They belong with the ambulance and should be used as dolleys to wheel patients who have been secured to their boards from one place to another. If a cot (rather than a board) is left with a patient at the hospital, either the usefulness of the ambulance is affected, or time will be wasted while the crew waits for the return of the cot. (If for any reason an ambulance is required to surrender a cot to the hospital, the crew should not wait for its return, but should head back to the scene immediately.)

DESIGN OF MASS CASUALTY BOARDS

Obviously, to be well prepared for an MCI requires about 100 extra long boards. This need not be the major expense that it seems. Inexpensive mass casualty boards can easily be made from sheets of 5/8-inch plywood.

The design of these boards has been carefully evolved and is based on experience. Notice that they differ from standard backboards in certain respects:

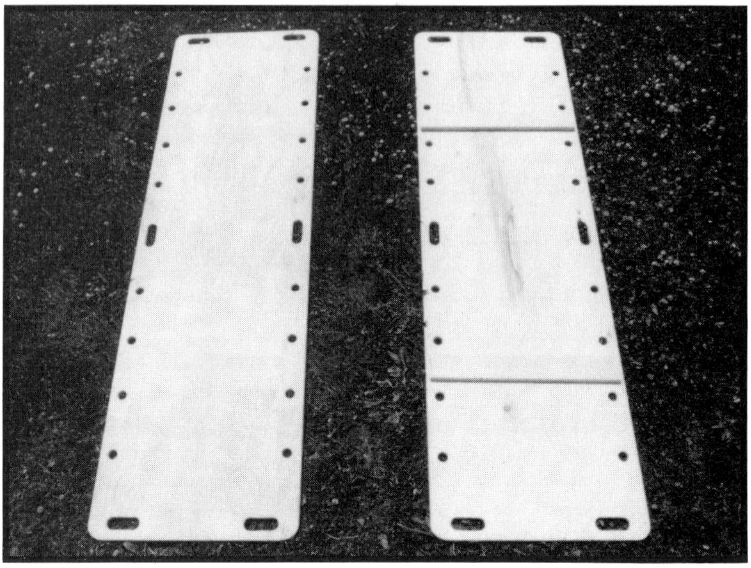

1. The boards are wider, so that arms and legs can easily be secured and will not hang off or project beyond the edge.
2. There is no "head" or "foot," eliminating time lost in getting the patient on the board the "right" way.
3. The cleats on the bottom run across the ends, instead of longitudinally, and they are spaced so the boards can rest steadily on the backs of school-bus seats.

STORING AND MOVING THE BOARDS

The storage, accessing, and moving of 100 wooden backboards presents some difficulties. Several methods are possible.

One is to store all 100 boards in the school-bus garage. A work force is then added to the call-up list to report to the garage and load the boards onto one of the school buses that is going to the scene. The advantage of this system is that the school buses are constantly maintained, so there will always be a vehicle capable of transporting the boards. There are drawbacks, however: the need for an additional work force, and the loss of time involved in handling so many boards as a separate step in the response plan.

Another method is to keep the boards on a van or truck ready to drive to the scene. This method has the advantage of cutting down on loading time and personnel. The initial expense can be overcome in part by using an old or surplus vehicle. However, since the vehicle sits idle for months at a time, the possibility exists that when the boards are needed, the vehicle won't start. (One service that had this problem at a drill dealt with it ingeniously: Instead of losing time by loading the boards onto another vehicle, they simply used a tow truck to tow the loaded van to the scene.)

A third method, possible in urban centers having large mass casualty bus ambulances, is to store the boards directly on these buses, which are constantly maintained and ready to go. This is not, however, a realistic method for small communities.

A fourth solution is to keep the boards on a trailer. If several response vehicles and the automobiles of key personnel have trailer hitches, there will always be a vehicle able to tow the trailer.

A fifth solution, and in our opinion the best, takes a regional approach. Every responding service has 10 mass casualty backboards, besides the 2 to 3 long boards routinely carried on each ambulance. These 10 boards can be stacked in the ambulance bay close to the back doors of the ambulance, ready for quick loading. Eight of the boards can be packaged in sets of 4 boards each; the other mass casualty equipment can be tied to the remaining 2 boards, so the entire complement of mass casualty supplies can be loaded quickly. This method has several obvious advantages. It spreads the financial responsibility for 100 backboards over the entire region; it allows for the best division of labor resulting in the least loss of time; and finally, the minute an ambulance reaches the scene, there are 12 or 13 boards ready for use.

IMMOBILIZING PATIENTS TO THE BOARDS

Before placing a patient on a board, the position that will be best for him must be determined. If the patient is unconscious, he may have to be secured in the coma position to preserve patency of the airway.

If the patient is conscious, not in respiratory distress, and C-spine injury is not suspected, use the procedure described here.

1. Move the patient to the normal anatomical position.
2. The patient can now be placed on the board or the board can be slid under the patient. A straddle lift or split litter may be used for this purpose; however, the latter may be excessively time-consuming. *Logrolling a multiple-trauma victim is inappropriate*. It promotes rotation of parts of the body, causing shifting stress on the limbs, chest, pelvis, and spine, which is contraindicated.

Experience has shown that it is best not to use buckled straps to immobilize patients to long boards. There will not be enough of them to go around; they will have to be removed before X rays can be taken; and their application often takes too much time. Instead, we recommend the use of cravats made from triangular bandages. They are cheap, can be quickly applied and swiftly cut off, and do not obstruct X rays. One mass casualty trunk should contain nothing but a large supply of prefolded cravats.

METHOD

1. Tie one cravat across the patient's chest, high on the sternum, as shown. Make sure the cravat is snug up under the armpits, and that it is tied tightly. This prevents the patient from slipping downward, while still permitting free chest rise during ventilation.

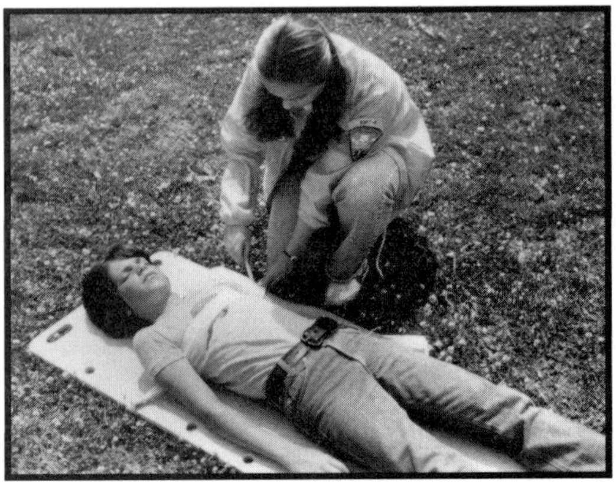

2. Tie the next cravat slightly below the patient's waist, passing it over the iliac crests rather than the soft abdomen. Both arms go under this one to keep them from falling off the board.

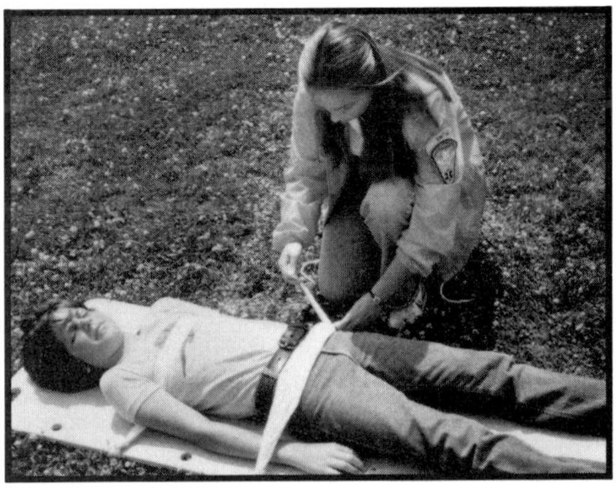

3. In order to prevent the natural outward rotation of the legs, tie both feet together. Place the cravat under the ankles, then bring the ends up on the outside of each leg. . . .

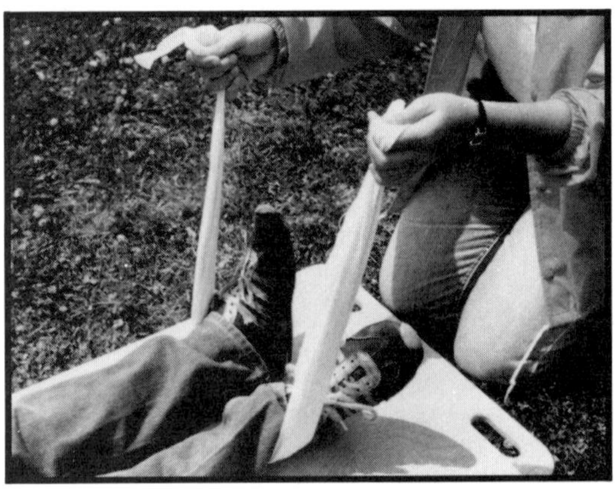

Pass the ends over the top of each foot, then between the feet. . . .

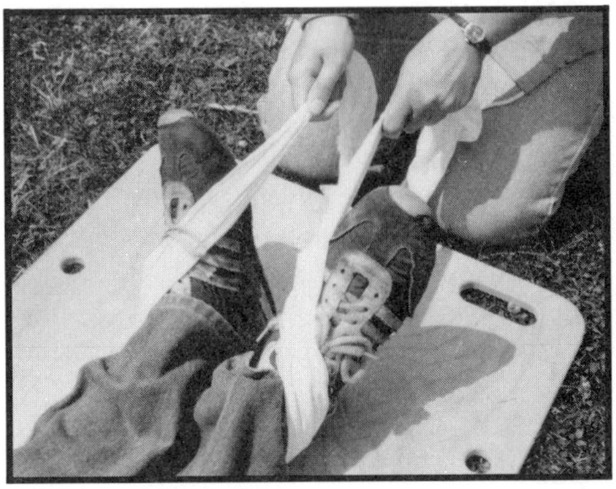

Finally bring the ends around the bottom of each foot, over the outer edge to the midline, and tie them together. . . .

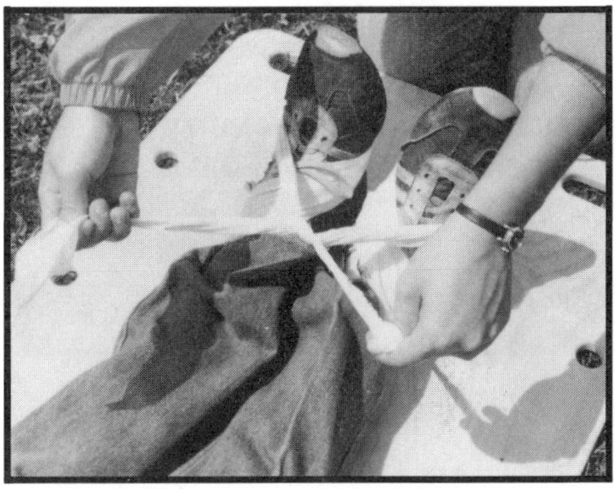

Finish off with a square knot or any other knot that does not travel.

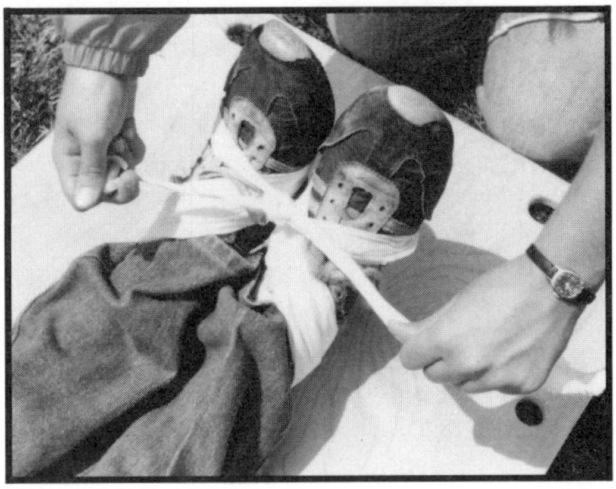

4. Fasten the legs to the board. This can be done by simply tying a cravat above the ankles.

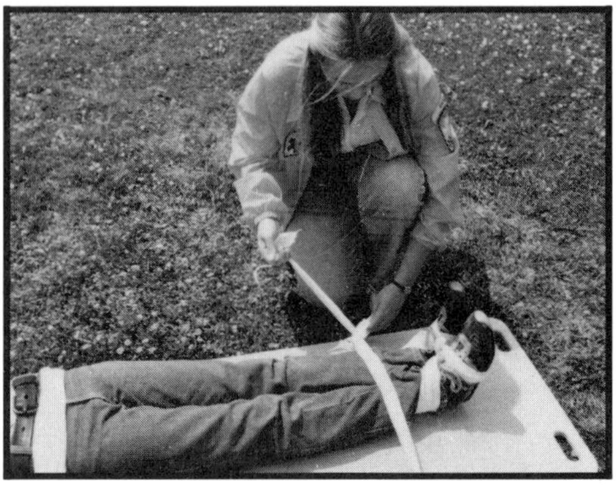

The basic system, using 4 cravats, can be completed in a few minutes—less time than it takes to determine the location of fractures—and it immobilizes and splints the entire body to the long board.

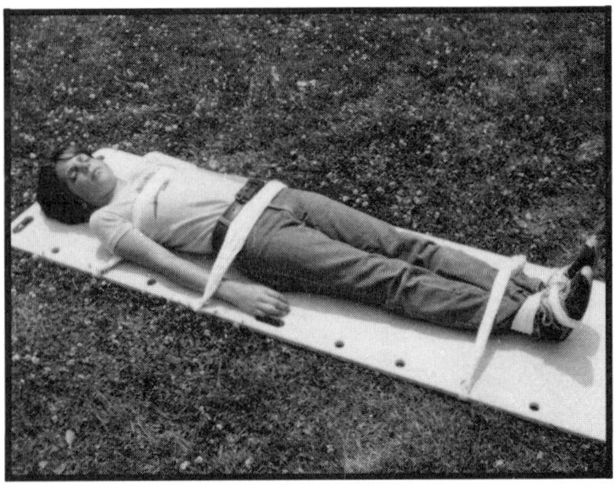

The technique can be abridged to use only three ties—(armpits, above the knees, and one to tie the feet) or expanded with a fifth cravat (armpits, below the waist, above the knees, above the ankles, and one to tie the feet).

Remember: once a patient is tied to a board, he should not be removed from it until definitive treatment is begun at the hospital. Ambulance crews should not attempt to take boards back to the scene with them; the boards will be recovered later.

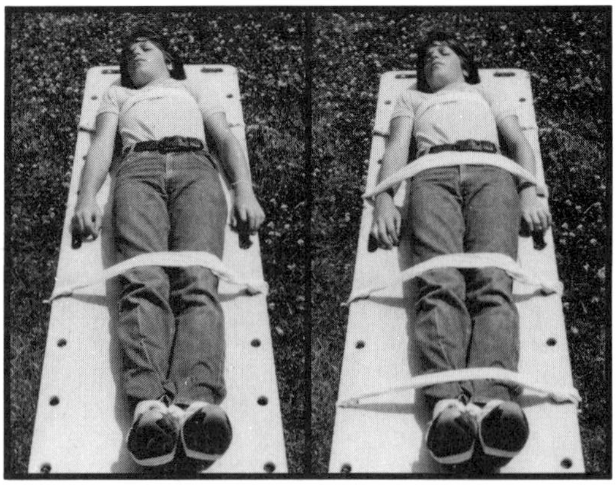

MULTIFRACTURE MODIFICATION

With a multiply injured patient, it may be desirable to avoid putting localized pressure on the legs by using the following device: Place a long wooden splint about 8 inches wide between the legs as shown. Pad the upper end of the splint at the patient's crotch. Run the cravat over this splint. Thus, the legs will be immobilized to the board but the bandage will not be pressing anterior to posterior. Some regions use T-shaped boards for this purpose, placing the crossbar of the T below the patient's feet for even greater stability.

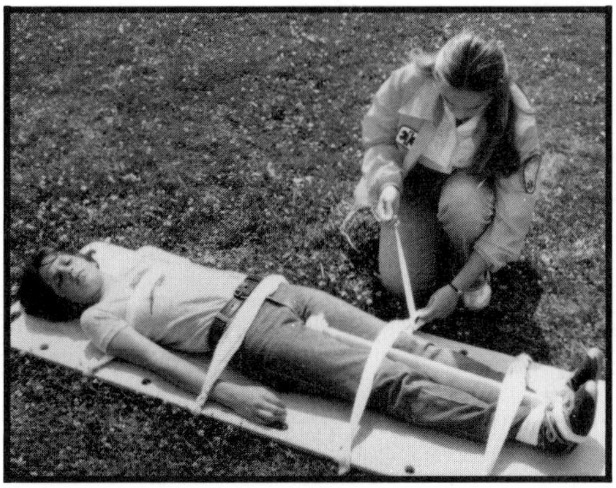

C-SPINE MODIFICATION

If a patient has a suspected cervical spine injury, start by applying hand traction and an extrication collar. Place the patient on the board while maintaining hand traction. Then follow the steps listed below. (Two EMTs will be needed for the procedure.)

1. Tie one cravat to each side of the board exactly even with the tops of the shoulders. Leave these cravats in place for future use.

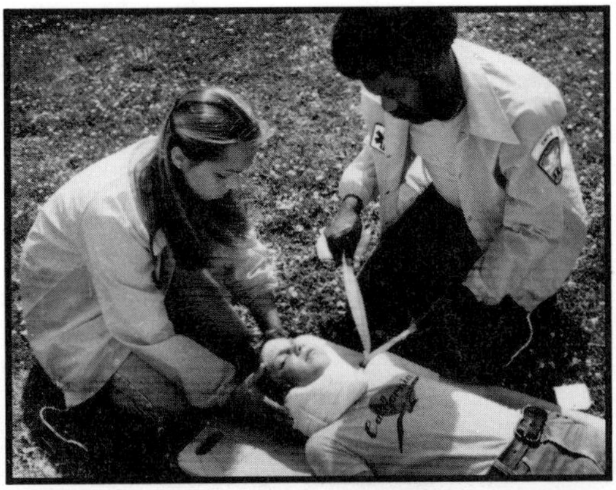

2. Make a blanket roll. (Practice will increase the ease with which you can roll a blanket into the proper length and shape.) Without jarring the EMT who is providing hand traction, place the blanket around the patient's head and along the shoulders as shown.

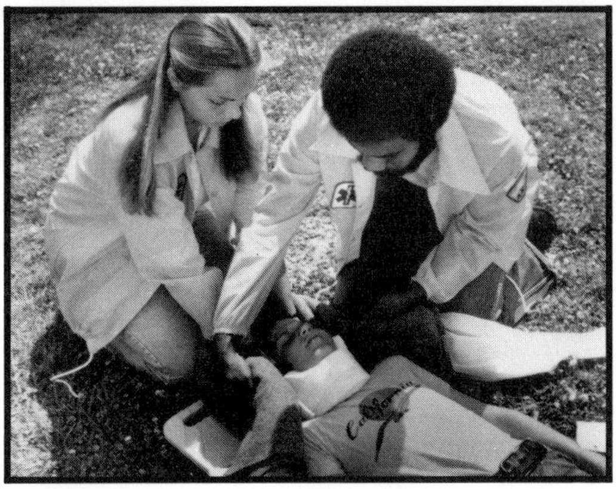

3. Take one of the cravats from Step 1 and pass it over the blanket and shoulder, across the upper sternum and the chest, and under the opposite armpit. Tie it to the board so that it is snug under the armpit and fairly tight.

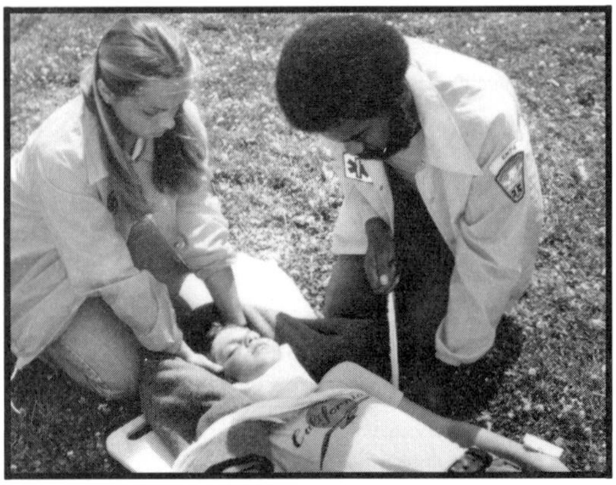

4. Repeat with the other cravat. Now an "X" has been formed across the chest, fastening the blanket roll and immobilizing the patient so he cannot slide up or down on the board.

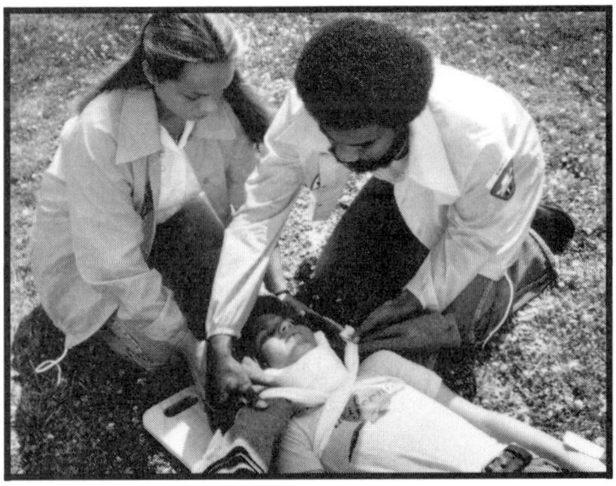

5. Remove hand traction and support the head and the blanket from the sides. Use 2 cravats to tie an "X" across the blanket and the forehead.

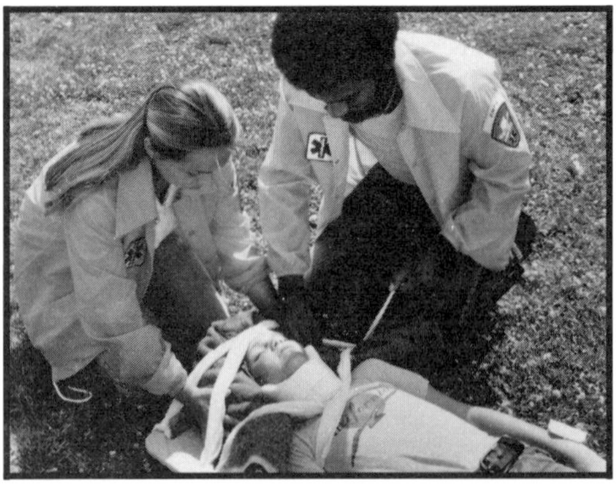

6. Add a waist tie passing over the arms. With a C-spine patient, this cravat must be tied snugly to prevent lateral motion of the torso. Proceed to the foot ties as in the basic method. The patient is now immobilized.

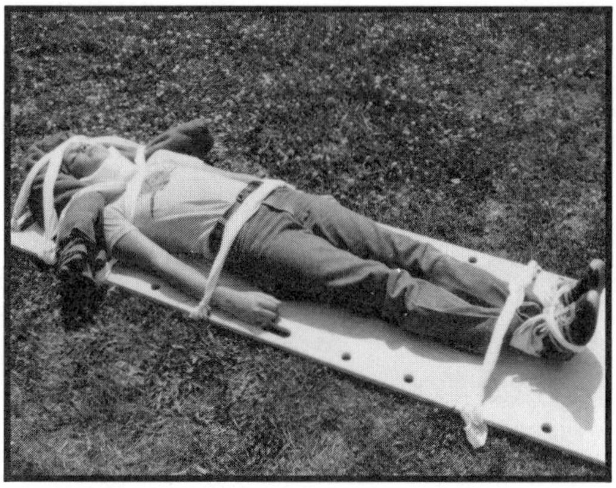

SPECIAL PROBLEMS

In a mass casualty situation it may be necessary to upend a board to evacuate a patient. The immobilization described above is adequate to support C-spine patients in an upright position. The "X" at the shoulders, tied tightly and snug into the armpits, will keep the upended patient from sliding toward his feet. (Patients should always be upended with the feet down.)

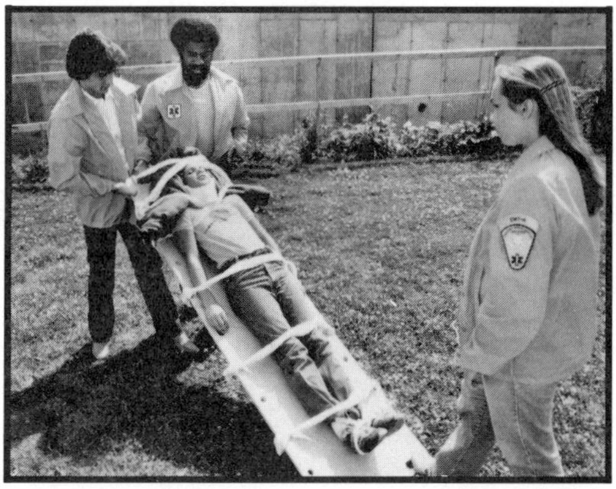

If injuries to the clavicle contraindicate an "X" over the chest, simply pass loops under the armpit and up over the same arm and the blanket as shown. The patient will be fully immobilized without any cravat crossing the clavicle.

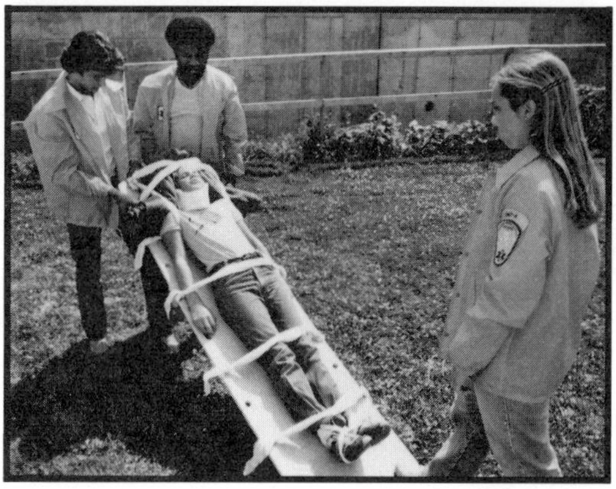

Where no spine injury is suspected and the patient will have to be upended, the fast tie method previously described should be supplemented by the addition of "X" straps at the shoulders and armpits.

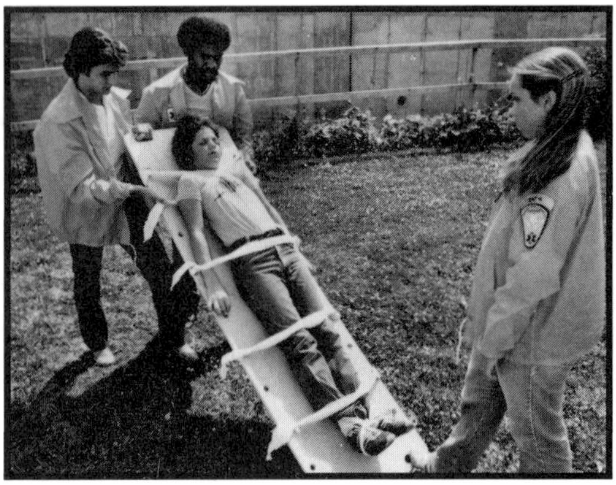

Or, use the single cravat across the chest and use 2 groin loops as shown.

Which method to use is determined by a quick inspection of the paths the cravats will follow, to detect possible underlying injury.

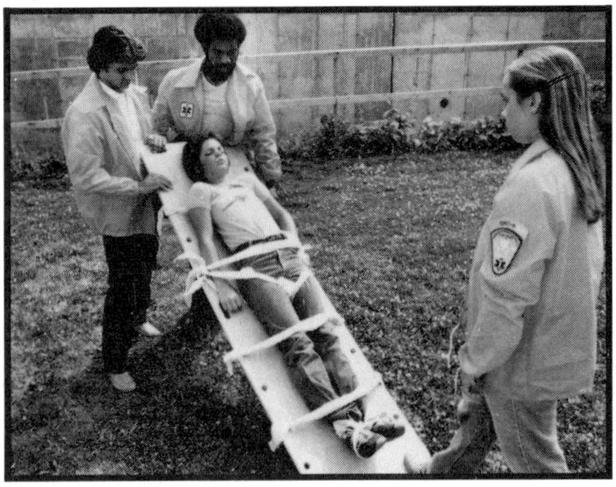

Although there usually won't be time to deal separately with individual injuries, an occasional patient may have a break that is impairing circulation distal to the injury (with resultant danger of ischemia and potential loss of the limb). It is sometimes possible to splint such a break separately. Evaluate the situation, taking into consideration loss of limb versus possible loss of life for someone else. If there is enough staff available in the field, and if treatment of the break will not delay the patient's transport, it may be possible to deal with the potential loss of limb.

In the event of a broken knee or elbow requiring splinting in flexion, flexible ladder splints or shapeable cardboard splints can be quick and effective, either in conjunction with the long board or separately.

Bandaging

In a mass casualty situation, the use of Kling, Con-form, and other roller bandages is time-consuming and often inappropriate. Triangular bandages, used as triangles or folded into cravats, represent a rapid method for bandaging any part of the body.

Training for mass casualty response should include practice in rapidly applying the bandages for all parts of the body. It is not enough to study diagrams of the methods for tying these bandages. All EMTs must have hands-on experience in making them. This practice is a required part of good mass casualty training.

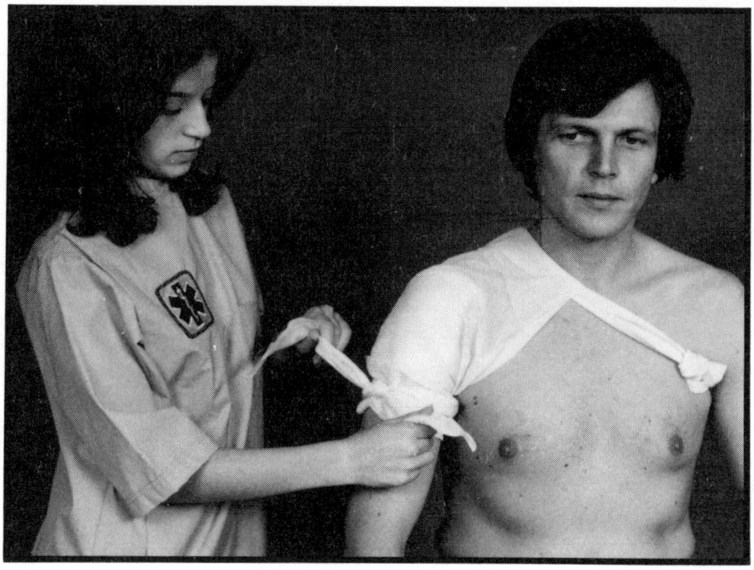

Chapter 9

CALL-UP PLANS: PERSONNEL AND EQUIPMENT

The call-up system is the cornerstone of a good mass casualty response plan. An effective call-up plan must meet 2 basic requirements:

1. The public must be able to access the plan; i.e., activate it.
2. The dispatcher must have a clear set of written instructions that detail whom to call and in what order.

Public Access

An area's normal EMS emergency telephone number (such as 911) should be the access number regardless of the quantity of victims—one, 30, or 100.

However, in a Mass Casualty Incident, people often call the police, the fire department, or the nearest hospital. The response plan must include a crossover procedure so that the information will be relayed to the proper EMS dispatcher. *Under no circumstances* should a caller with information about a disaster be told, "You have to call the central dispatcher. Hang up and dial 911." Instead, whoever receives the call—be it a police officer, a firefighter, or a switchboard operator at a local hospital—should take down the information and relay it to EMS Dispatch. As a part of the plan, all agencies that might possibly be called with such a report should be taught what information to ask for and how to relay it promptly and concisely.

Dispatch Protocols

It has been our experience that call-up procedures are generalized and flexible while response procedures are very specific. *It should be the other way around.* Call-up procedures, specified in complete detail, should be the only rigid element in the entire plan.

Protocols establishing whom to call and in what order should be carefully worked out in advance. These protocols should be written out, word-for-word. It is only human to become nervous when a disaster is being reported. The margin for error is greatly reduced if the dispatcher is not required to make decisions, but only to follow a predetermined call-up procedure. Therefore, the instructions should not say, "Alert fire department," but should tell the dispatcher exactly what words to use. In this way, the dispatcher simply reads out what he or she sees. All instructions should be included, such as which buttons to push and when to push them.

There should be 2 sets of initial procedures for Dispatch to follow, depending on whether the report is confirmed or unconfirmed.

CONFIRMED CALLS

A *confirmed* call is one that comes from any uniformed responder—a policeman or a firefighter, for instance—or from any known, reliable, and responsible source such as the commander of a local military base, the head of the airport, the head ranger of a park, or any known member of a government agency. Dispatch may want to check the authenticity of the call by telephoning the agency in question for verification; however, this should not be done until the initial call-up has gone out. If the call was a hoax, the responders can easily be recalled at this point; if it was not, valuable time would have been lost by checking before beginning the call-up.

A report may also be considered confirmed if a number of independent, unrelated calls come in from the public telling of the same incident.

UNCONFIRMED CALLS

An *unconfirmed* call is any call coming from the public. An unconfirmed call will be either confirmed or denied by the first uniformed responder on the scene. He will also provide an estimate of the number of victims.

The difference between the procedures for an unconfirmed and a confirmed call is: *local* resources are called up on the unconfirmed report; *regional* resources are called up when confirmation of the report is received. Each of these possibilities will be given separate consideration.

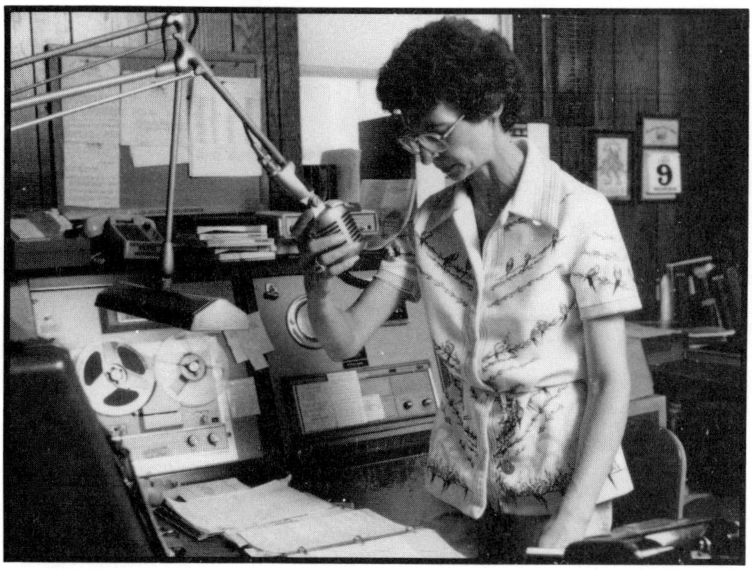

Unconfirmed Call-Up: Local Resources

The following is a sample of the protocols for an unconfirmed mass casualty.

1. On police frequency transmit:
   "This is KDP429–Central Dispatch. Police Units 20 and 40 respond to an unconfirmed signal '1000' at *Smithtown Highway, between Exits 4 and 5*, north lane."
2. Activate fire department tone alert and transmit:
   "KDT-130 to all Weston firemen and rescue personnel with a signal '1000'. All fire and rescue personnel report to your firehouses."
3. Activate EMS tone alert and transmit:
   "KDT-130 to all Weston ambulance personnel with a signal '1000'. All ambulance personnel report with turnout gear, crash kits, and tone alert receivers to headquarters."
4. Call Lincoln Hospital Emergency Department (555-3533) and tell them: "This is Weston Emergency Communications. We have an unconfirmed signal '1000.'" Indicate its nature.
5. Page EMS Executive Dave Moore. Page code AWLL. State type and location of incident.
6. Page EMS Assistant Executive Bill Rogers. Page code AWSL. State type and location of incident.
7. Call the Department of Public Works (555-7997). Tell them to send 4 trucks to scene.
8. Call Bob's Towing (555-1326). Send 2 tow trucks to scene.
9. Call school-bus garage (555-2324). Send 5 buses to scene.

Note that this set of protocols calls for the police to be notified first. In some areas, it may be more effective to send the fire department first. For example, if a fire department has many neighborhood stations with staff always on duty, they may be able to reach the scene more quickly than the police. This decision can only be made on a local basis—but it should be made ahead of time and be written into the call-up instructions. Do not expect the dispatcher or anyone else to make that decision while an incident is in progress; this will only cause a loss of time and may lead to unsound decisions made in haste.

After the first uniformed responder confirms the incident and estimates the number of injured, additional dispatchers are called to help throughout the rest of the emergency. (Note: If funds are available, tone-alert receivers for all dispatchers are a good investment. With just one call, EMS Dispatch would be able to contact several dispatchers to assist in the MCI.)

The most efficient call-up method is a *fan-out* system. Under this system, EMS Dispatch makes one call to the police dispatcher, who then proceeds to call up police resources according to a prearranged plan. EMS Dispatch then makes similar calls to the fire department dispatcher and to the near-hospital operator. Each of these dispatchers then calls up his own resources. This system leaves EMS Dispatch free to handle communications with the incident site.

If such a fan-out system is not possible, your plan must provide for the *early* summoning of more dispatchers to handle the communications problems that will arise.

Ideally, the EMS radio setup should be arranged so that once everyone is alerted, all can go to a common frequency for updates on the incident. Even if radio dialers or segregated frequencies exist for each hospital, there should be a common emergency frequency. If all service departments and hospitals can hear Control describing what personnel and equipment will be needed, radio communications can be minimized, increasing efficiency and saving time—an obvious advantage.

Confirmed Call-Up: Regional Resources

When a Mass Casualty Incident is confirmed, the regional resources are called in. At the end of this section, there is a continuation of the call-up procedures begun here. However, before these protocols can be set forth, some discussion of whom to call and why may be helpful.

Hospitals. The near hospitals are now notified that a confirmed incident has taken place involving about 60 patients. If the hospitals had not activated their disaster response plans upon receipt of the unconfirmed report, they would do so now. (Whether to activate on an unconfirmed report is subject to each hospital's protocols.)

When the patient count is received, the near hospitals will, by prearranged plan, notify the far hospitals of the situation and tell them how many patients they can expect. This effectively breaks down the job of notifying *all* hospitals into several smaller tasks.

Nearby fire departments and rescue crews. Fire and rescue personnel will be called by EMS Dispatch or by the fire department as dictated by the fire control officer. (Regional plans must provide for at least one backup unit for each department to cover local areas, just as with ambulances that respond.) More firefighters will be needed at the scene than will be required to fight any fires. Extra firefighters represent a structured, disciplined work force that can undertake a wide range of assignments at the scene.

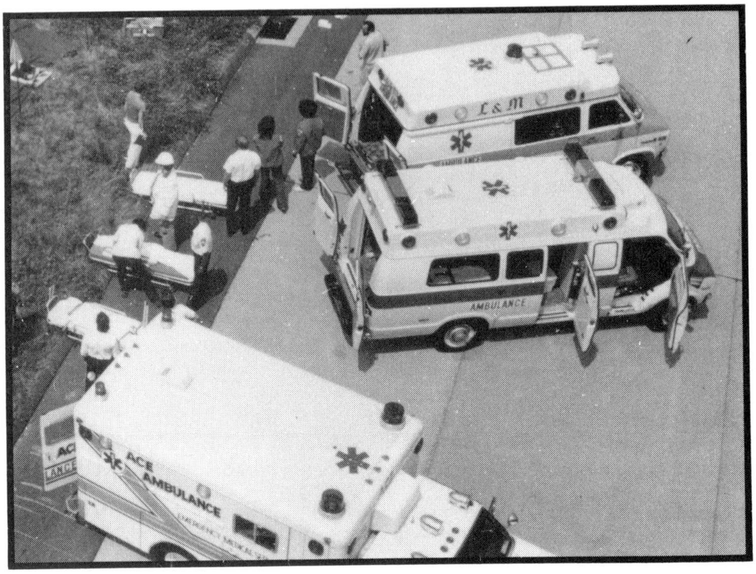

Ambulances. Your plan should have arranged access for up to 10 specified ambulances besides the on-call ambulance that was sent out on the unconfirmed report. The total number of ambulances, local and regional, should be 11, one of which will remain at the scene to serve as an on-site control and communications center. The other 10 will be used for transporting patients. The number 10 was not selected at random. Experience has shown that 10 ambulances will sustain a continuous cycle of delivery to the near hospitals. In other words, just as the tenth ambulance is pulling out with its quota of stabilized victims, the first one will be returning from its trip, ready to pick up 2 more patients. Since this cycle generally coincides with the amount of time required in the field to stabilize patients for transport, each patient will spend a minimum of time waiting for an ambulance.

If the incident involves 60 patients, and 2 can travel in each ambulance, then each ambulance will have to make 3 trips. Some ambulances will make even fewer trips since some or most of the Greens can be transported by bus.

Obviously, calling up 10 ambulances from other towns in a region reduces the ability of each town to provide normal emergency care for its citizens. Therefore, regional response plans must include backup systems to cover the responding towns while the MCI is absorbing area ambulances and personnel. Ambulance-summoning plans should be worked out regionally so that each town sending ambulances is properly covered. The plan should ensure that the covering ambulance is not assumed to be covering other towns also, and that it won't be summoned to the scene.

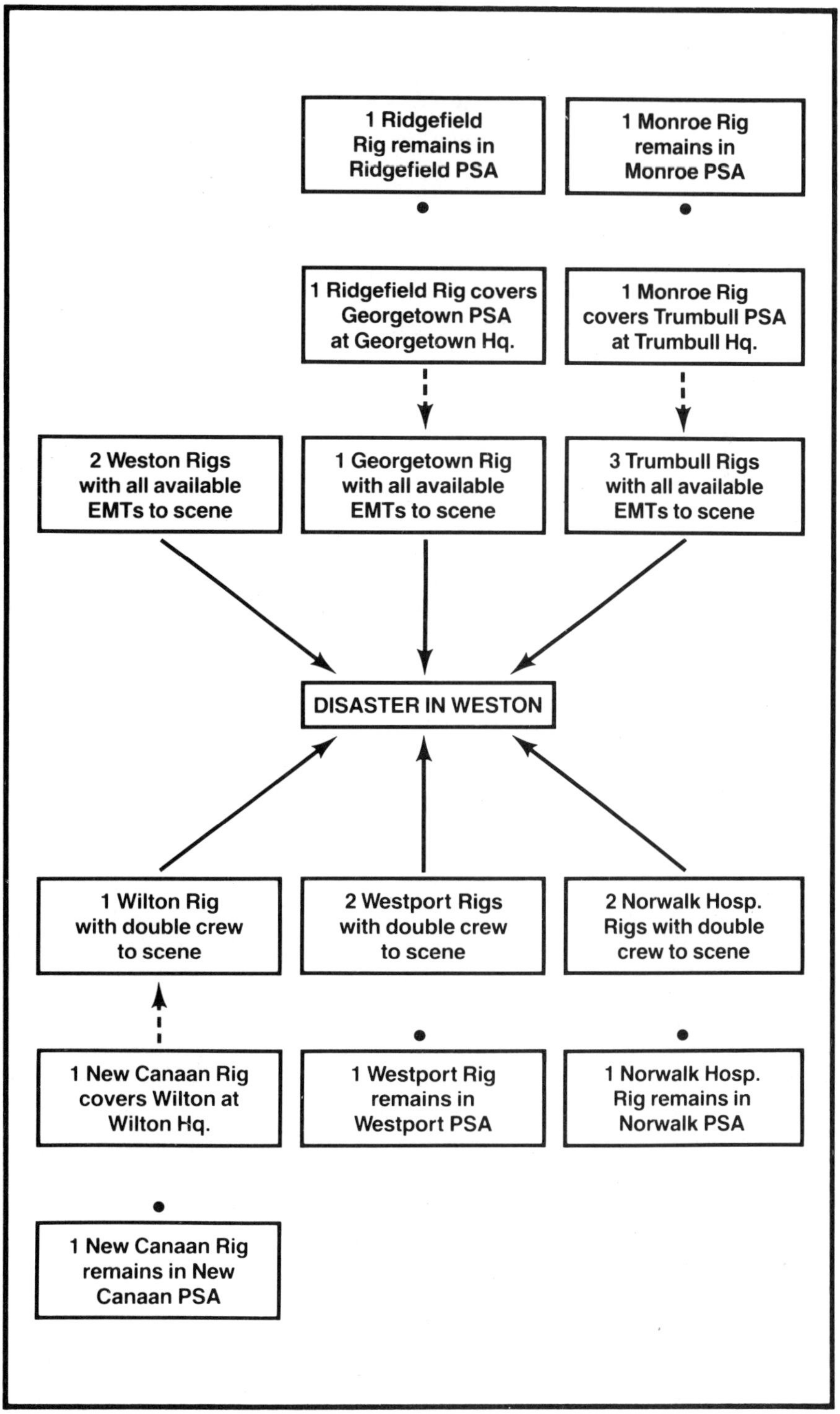
1 Ridgefield Rig remains in Ridgefield PSA
1 Monroe Rig remains in Monroe PSA
1 Ridgefield Rig covers Georgetown PSA at Georgetown Hq.
1 Monroe Rig covers Trumbull PSA at Trumbull Hq.
2 Weston Rigs with all available EMTs to scene
1 Georgetown Rig with all available EMTs to scene
3 Trumbull Rigs with all available EMTs to scene
DISASTER IN WESTON
1 Wilton Rig with double crew to scene
2 Westport Rigs with double crew to scene
2 Norwalk Hosp. Rigs with double crew to scene
1 New Canaan Rig covers Wilton at Wilton Hq.
1 Westport Rig remains in Westport PSA
1 Norwalk Hosp. Rig remains in Norwalk PSA
1 New Canaan Rig remains in New Canaan PSA

The selection of covering squads should be based neither upon intercommunity relationships, nor on considerations of distance alone. It must also be based on each squad's manpower, the ability of each squad to summon its members, their levels of training, and *travel times*—not distances. The consideration should always be, "Once we've called them, how long will it take them to get here, and what can they bring?"

Each service should also have a plan that indicates its procedure when summoned to an MCI in a *neighboring* town. The exact response may be different for *each* nearby community. All ambulances from one town may be sent to the disaster site, and the dispatcher may then summon one ambulance from another community to cover. For a different nearby service, the response agreed upon might be to send all but one ambulance, keeping the one to cover the local community. The key element in ambulance summoning is *regional preplanning*.

The diagram below shows how one type of covering plan works. Upon verification of a Mass Casualty Incident, ambulances from towns immediately surrounding the disaster area are summoned and move to the site. The ambulances in the ring surrounding the responding group cover the regular EMS needs in their own area as well as in the areas that are uncovered.

All regional volunteer ambulances should be double-crewed; this should be specified in the call-up protocols. EMS services having one crew always on duty should not wait for extra personnel to arrive; the extra personnel can gather at headquarters and come to the scene by car or by bus. (This bus should be on the call-up list.)

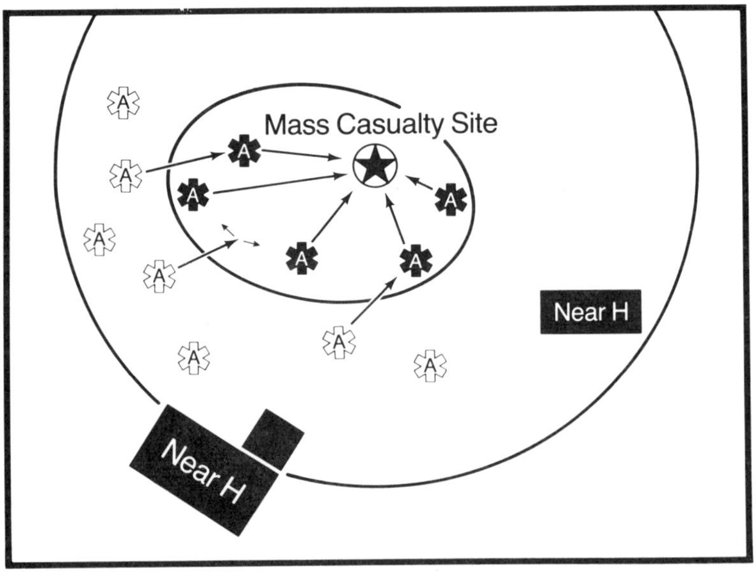

A tone-alert paging system is of great value in a mass casualty situation; it saves the time that would be lost in telephoning personnel separately. If key EMS leadership personnel have tone-alert receivers, precise pager code instructions should appear on the dispatcher's call-up checklist, e.g., "Page Dave Moore. Pager code: AWLL."

By prearrangement, key town officers—the Mayor and any other personnel agreed upon—should be notified soon after the incident is confirmed. The required names and telephone numbers should be on the dispatcher's checklist.

ADDITIONAL REQUIRED PERSONNEL

Bus and tow truck drivers. Before the MCI is confirmed, 2 tow trucks and 4 or 5 buses should be called to the scene. After confirmation, more buses may be dispatched if the conditions warrant it. Protocols for buses should include provisions for the following: drivers to carry EMTs from their stations to the scene; drivers to transport Green patients to hospitals; drivers to carry relatives of victims to hospitals (see Chapter 12). In inclement weather, buses can be used as heated collecting stations. Provision should be made in advance for 3 or 4 additional buses for this purpose, if necessary. All drivers should know where to get their buses; they should be provided with keys to garages, if necessary; and they should know where they are to report (that is, to the scene, to the ambulance headquarters, or elsewhere).

The local school-bus company is the obvious source for both buses and drivers; if this is not a viable option, other plans should be made in advance. (For example, firefighters may be trained to drive the buses.)

The Department of Public Works. It may be necessary to sand icy roads and operate bulldozers or backhoes. In the course of some rescue efforts, large objects must be moved. In a building collapse, for instance, parts of the building may need to be lifted from possible survivors. Local construction companies may also be able to supply men and equipment for this job; make arrangements with them ahead of time.

Specialty groups. Depending on the terrain, an area may have any or all of the following: riding clubs, ski clubs, snowshoe clubs, snowmobile clubs, toboggan clubs, scuba clubs, boating or canoe clubs, and mountain search and rescue teams, members of which are familiar with local geography.

Any of these groups, if briefed ahead of time and taught what will be expected of them, can be helpful in gaining access to areas where vehicles cannot go. They have the necessary clothing and supplies and are trained in their use.

It should be the job of the local and regional Civil Preparedness organizations to locate, instruct, and inventory these groups, so that Central Dispatch will know how they can be most easily and rapidly summoned, if they are needed. This inventory should be corrected every 6 months by telephoning the head of each organization. Update him or her on the mass casualty response plan and obtain revised records of membership.

The Red Cross. These people are experienced in disaster work and should be able to help in many ways: supplying food, bandages and other materials, locating shelter for relatives of victims, etc.

Food personnel. If a Red Cross chapter is not readily available, a local restauranteur may agree to provide food during an operation that seems likely to go on for an extended period. If so, he should be on the call-up list. As an alternative, members of local organizations (Kiwanis, Rotary, etc.) can be briefed ahead of time so they will know where food and supplies can be obtained and how a kitchen can be set up off-site. (Local organizations can also provide willing hands to help with the many nonmedical, nonrescue elements of the situation.)

Military personnel. If there is a military base nearby, its personnel should be a part of the response plan. The military has supplies that many towns cannot afford—large tents and ambulance buses, for instance—as well as the trained personnel to operate this equipment.

Extra ambulances. Though most MCIs can be dealt with using the basic 11 ambulances called for in this demonstration, there may be occasions when more ambulances will be required. Plans should include a way to call up an additional 10 ambulances, complete with covering ambulances for the responding towns.

Fuel. All vehicles will probably need refueling. If it has its own pumps, the Department of Public Works may be able to fill this need. If not, have a centrally located gas station available for use. (Provide for diesel fuel if it will be necessary.) If distances are great, it may be advisable to make arrangements with stations on the perimeter of the area as well. Make sure that some responsible person has a key or can gain access to the pumps at any time, day or night. Station owners or operators should be on the call-up list.

Continuation of a Sample Call-Up

Now that the need for extra personnel and equipment has been explained, we can go on with the call-up procedures.

When the call is confirmed, the following checklist, adapted to meet local needs, should be followed.

10. Call Mayor Renzulli (555-2397).
11. Call Head of Civil Preparedness, Jane Cleese (555-2999).
12. Call Lincoln Hospital (555-3533). Tell them the signal "1000" has been confirmed. Report the estimated number of patients.
13. Call Smithfield EMS for 2 ambulances (555-1246).
14. Call Johnson County EMS for 3 ambulances (555-1913).
15. Call Lincoln County EMS; tell them you have a confirmed signal "1000" and need their 5 ambulances.
16. On the county fire band, call up county control and have them dispatch Smithfield, West Lake, and Thomasville for an MCI.
17. Call Red Cross director, Clara Syms (555-1113).
18. Call Salvation Army director, Bill Andrews (555-1173).
19. Call Santossi's Service Station, owner Bill Santossi (555-6117). Tell him to open his station for a disaster in progress.
20. Etc.

Supplies and Equipment

Basic supplies. As part of the response plan, each ambulance service should have an inventory of basic supplies to meet the initial needs of patients in the field. These supplies should be packed in marked footlockers or trunks. One of the trunks should contain nothing but dressings and triangular bandages, prefolded into

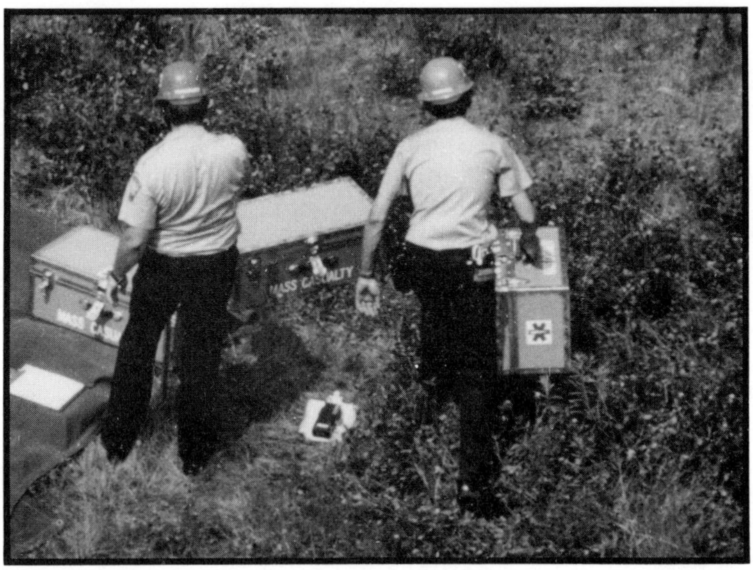

cravats. Another should contain triage tags and plenty of writing implements, oxygen masks, and flashlights.

IV supplies. The inventory should include 100 IV sets. One hundred containers of IV fluids are also required. The difficulty is that IV fluids have a short shelf life and must be used before the expiration date on each container. There are several ways to deal with this problem.

1. Keep 100 containers on hand; when they near the expiration date, throw them away and replace them with fresh ones. This system has the drawback of being wasteful, but it will ensure that fresh IV fluids will always be available.
2. Keep 100 containers on hand; when they begin to approach the end of their shelf life, rotate them with a local hospital. The hospital, which will be able to use the IV solutions quickly, can trade them for fresher containers.
3. Do not try to keep large quantities on hand; instead, make arrangements for the nearest hospital to deliver 100 fresh containers to the scene promptly when an incident occurs. Arrangements must include replenishing the hospital's supply from farther hospitals.

However, even with 100 fresh containers on hand, it is probable that supplies will run out. In all, as many as 200 containers, and the corresponding number of IV sets and catheters, will probably be needed. Therefore, the response plan must include a way to locate more IV supplies.

If there is a large surgical supply house nearby, the problem may be solved. Usually, however, the best method is to get more IV supplies from an outlying hospital—preferably one so far away that it is not likely to be heavily involved in the disaster. The distant hospital can transport the required supplies to a near hospital (via local ambulance or police squad car), and that hospital, in turn, can give the supplies to an ambulance crew returning to the field.

Where IV teams are dispatched to the field, they should *bring their own supplies* and be responsible for replacing them.

Whole blood will also be in short supply; however, this is a hospital problem and, as such, is not covered here.

Bandages. Additional bandages will probably also be required. The Red Cross is one possible source.

Oxygen. Know where to locate a portable oxygen refiller that is available 24 hours a day. A hospital is the most likely source. A nearby medical gas supply company may also be able to help. Arrangements can be made for bulk tanks of oxygen to be delivered to the scene for refilling portable tanks, or for a "cascade" filling system, or for a portable oxygen truck.

Blankets. These can be obtained from the Red Cross or the Salvation Army. Prearrange for extra blankets to be taken to the site. Have on hand 100 disposable plastic drop cloths for use over blankets in inclement weather. An exposed blanket acts as a wick, pulling every drop of moisture in to the patient's body. A plastic drop cloth will prevent this. Be sure the cloth is kept well away from the patient's mouth and nose, of course.

Backpacks. In areas covering remote wilderness terrain, backpacks capable of holding all necessary supplies must be available. In fact, in these areas it may be wise to store all supplies in such packs. This will save time if an incident does occur in rough terrain. Should an incident occur in an area that's easily reached by vehicles, the supplies can still be transported to the scene in the packs, and easily carried about the scene as required. If the town cannot afford to supply packs, it may be possible to make arrangements with local backpacking groups for the donation of the necessary equipment.

Lighting supplies. Plenty of flashlights and fresh batteries must be available for nighttime or underground incidents. Remember, too, that the rescue trucks from local and neighboring fire departments carry lights powerful enough to illuminate the scene.

Communication supplies. For radio communication, the regular line-of-duty equipment to be found in ambulances and police vehicles will serve. For public announcements, use the electric megaphones available on most fire trucks. Segregated walkie-talkies for key EMS leadership personnel can be very helpful, if the community can afford the cost.

Hospital phone lines. During an MCI, the hospital switchboard may be so flooded with calls that it goes under. When this occurs, getting official communication in and out of the Emergency Department and hospital command center becomes impossible. This problem is easily resolved by installing several unlisted outside lines that go directly into the Emergency Department without passing through the switchboard. These "hot lines" can be profitably used on a daily basis by EMS services for call-in and ALS communication. (If one phone number is withheld even from EMS, it will always be free for the Emergency Department to call *out* on.) Some hospitals have put similar lines in the administration offices. These unlisted numbers are for hospital personnel to call in on, to confirm that they are needed when an incident is reported on the public radio and television.

Extra supplies. It is almost part of the definition of an MCI that there will be insufficient materials on hand to deal with the situation. You will probably run out of backboards, IV fluid and sets, bandages, and portable oxygen. Therefore, a good response plan will include instructions on where to go to get more supplies.

Conclusion

Routine MCI dispatching should be rigidly followed upon receipt of a call. Special needs, as noted by Control, are relayed to the dispatcher. A detailed, tab-indexed guide book will enable the dispatcher to locate personnel or items requested promptly. This guidebook must be tested and updated continuously. Remember: personnel, equipment, and supplies that are unsummoned, summoned too late, or not located, *don't arrive*—and, therefore, *don't exist*.

Chapter 10

PROPER UTILIZATION OF EMTs, PHYSICIANS, AND OTHERS

Utilization of EMTs

Owing to differing levels of training, the degree of meaningful intervention that the EMT is able to provide differs across the nation. In some regions, EMTs have Paramedic capabilities; in others, EMTs are limited to Basic Life Support; while in many regions, there is a mixture—some EMTs limited to BLS, while others are at the EMT-Intermediate or the EMT-P level.

Many MCI victims can be stabilized in the field with such BLS skills as putting the patient in the coma position, achieving slight extension of the head, using direct pressure to stop hemorrhage, and providing oxygen support. However, it is important to remember that most victims of an MCI will be suffering from multiple trauma. This means that most deaths will be due to shock (secondary to hypovolemia) and hypoxia. (Though few who survive the original insult die of external hemorrhage, many deaths can be attributed to intra-abdominal bleeding, hemothorax, etc.)

It follows that the EMTs who will be best able to treat MCI victims are those who have ALS training and can provide meaningful intervention for shock, respiratory problems, and bleeding—both internal and external. In order to stabilize a severe multiple-trauma victim, a responder must be able to apply anti-shock trousers, intubate and/or obturate, and start IVs.

It is of critical importance, therefore, that the varying levels of EMTs be properly deployed. In short, it is foolish to have BLS responders tending the victims while ALS personnel drive ambulances or carry patients about.

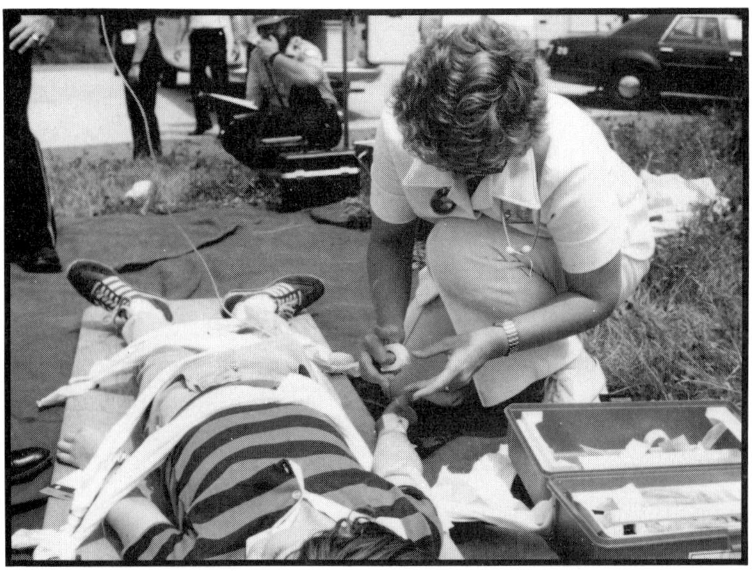

In areas where all EMTs are at the ALS level, there is no difficulty arranging for proper utilization of personnel. Similarly, in areas where only BLS responders are available, there is no deployment problem. (In the latter instance, it *is* necessary to ensure the rapid arrival of IV-, respiratory-, and MAST-trained teams that will treat patients at the collecting station.)

It is in areas where mixed levels of EMT responders are available, that thought must be given to proper utilization of skills.

NEED FOR A DISCIPLINED LABOR FORCE

Basic to the proper utilization of personnel is the availability of a large force of disciplined workers for activities that do not involve any medical knowledge (particularly carrying patients—a job requiring 4 people if your responders are not to collapse from physical exhaustion). As has been said elsewhere in this book, we assume that the regional fire departments will provide just such a force. An analysis of MCIs shows that if ignition occurs, and the firefighters are occupied with the fire, there will be more deaths and fewer patients requiring treatment. If there is no ignition, the firefighters will be available to help with the greater number of severely injured survivors. An exception to this generalization in my personal experience, was the Danbury Prison fire. There, our rescue and transportation efforts were slowed by the fact that a fire was burning *elsewhere* in the prison. We suffered from a lack of that disciplined work crew usually supplied by the firefighters—a fact that emphasizes the importance of such assistance.

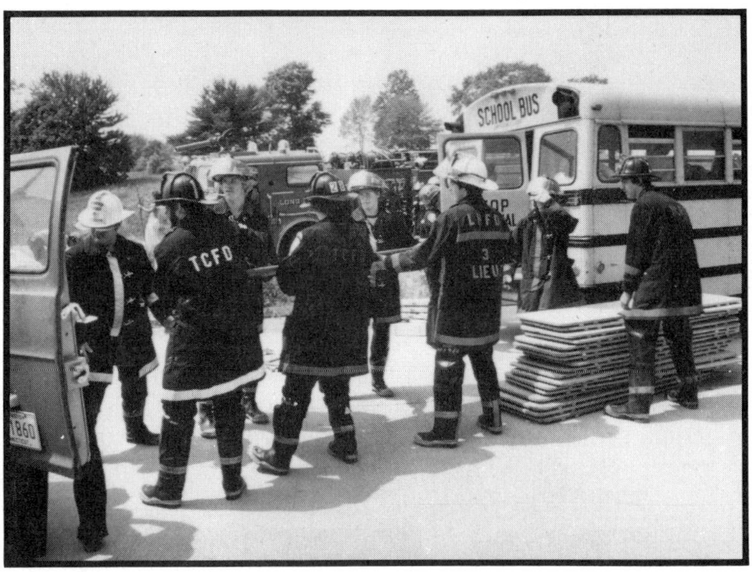

If there are insufficient firefighters to form a labor force, some other source of strong, disciplined personnel and good drivers must be found. Some areas may be able to make arrangements with college athletic teams, which are composed of healthy, responsible young people. Local clubs and organizations may also be contacted for this purpose. As a general rule, it is unwise to rely upon the police for this job; they almost always are completely involved with crowd and traffic control.

In areas where *all* ambulance responders, including the drivers, are EMTs, firefighters should be assigned to drive the ambulances, freeing the EMTs for work at the field.

Chronological Run-Through

Returning to our school bus example, we will go through the incident step by step, showing how the responders can best be utilized at each stage of events.

When the first 2 ambulances arrive, 2 or 3 of the crew board the bus and begin doing the primary survival scan. Another crew member assumes the job of Acting Control. The patients are not ready to come off the bus yet (except for those categorized Green) so there is no need for a Triage or Transportation Officer. Acting Control arranges for the placement of salvage covers for the collecting station.

Of the next 3 to 5 EMTs who arrive, one will take on the job of Acting Triage Officer, and one, the job of Acting Transportation Officer, until the actual officers arrive at the scene. The Acting Triage Officer organizes the process of getting the Green patients to the collecting station, if it is ready.

The Acting Transportation Officer takes on the job of deploying incoming personnel. Soon afterward, the actual officers should begin to arrive and take over their functions. By now, there should be a number of EMTs also. If early-arriving ALS personnel were assigned to the bus and to clearing patients off the bus, they should be relieved by BLS personnel. As they are replaced, these ALS personnel should be sent to the collecting station to begin treatment. The only exception to this should be one or 2 ALS-EMTs who remain on the bus to treat trapped patients.

Doctors, nurses, and EMTs from other areas, who are not familiar with local plans and protocols, should also be sent to the collecting station. These people will be very useful in treating patients, but would be likely to cause confusion in any other role.

When the Triage Officer arrives, the Acting Triage Officer should remain at the collecting station with the patients categorized Green. At this stage, the Triage Officer will be at the doors to the bus, triaging patients as they are unloaded. When enough patients have arrived at the collecting station to require his presence, the Triage Officer will return there to categorize the remaining patients.

Most of the EMTs who arrived initially were directed to the bus for primary survival scan. When the scan has been performed on all survivors, patient assessment and unloading begin. As each patient is unloaded from the bus, he is carried to the collecting station by 4 people—3 firefighters and the EMT who did the assessment. The EMT reports directly to the Triage Officer on his findings, minimizing the confusion and error that could result if messages were passed back and forth by intermediaries. As soon as his report is made, the EMT returns to the bus for another patient.

Meanwhile, because no patients are ready for transport yet, the Transportation Officer tells the arriving ambulances where to park and what to unload.

(A word about unloading. Commonly, the first ambulance crews to arrive begin to unload their equipment immediately. This is an error. Personnel at this point are most urgently needed on the bus doing primary survival scan. Equipment can be unloaded as necessary, before the ambulances begin rounds to the hospitals. Only when enough personnel have arrived to care for the patients should any crewmen be directed to spend time unloading. If sufficient firemen are present, they can be used for this work, freeing more EMTs for survey and assessment.)

A second error often committed by ambulance crews is to remain possessively with their ambulance. Instead, they should immediately report to the Transportation Officer for assignments on the field.

Note: When an ambulance leaves for the hospital, someone from its crew should be on board. This will be discussed later.

Areas of Activity

Notice that there are 4 areas of activity, and that they are filled in sequence as EMTs arrive.

Area 1: the bus. Early arrivals board the bus and begin to survey and assess the patients. By the time these steps are approaching completion, more EMTs have arrived, providing personnel for the second area of activity.

Area 2: transport from the bus to the collecting station. As the number of patients who are ready to go to the collecting station increases, the number of arriving responders also increases, so the process of carrying patients to the station can begin. Eight to 12 responders are enough to form a continuous chain between the bus and the collecting station.

Area 3: the collecting station. As soon as they can be released from other jobs, ALS personnel come to the collecting station to treat accumulating patients. The first 4 who reach the collecting station remain there as row monitors. They do not return for more patients. The next responders to arrive at the scene should be directed to the collecting station. Of all 4 areas of activity, the collecting station is the most labor-intensive. The more personnel available to treat patients, the greater the salvage rate will be. (Note: The focus of care should be Red patients first, then Yellow, Yellow Prime, and finally Green. Triage is not just to determine transportation priorities, but treatment priorities too.)

Notice that, at each step of the way, as more patients are ready to move to the next field of activity, more responders will have arrived to take care of that process. Only when all 3 of these fields of activity are sufficiently filled should activity begin in Area 4.

Area 4: transportation. The near hospitals will need time to implement their disaster plans, so there is little point in rushing patients to them prematurely. There are, of course, exceptions to this general rule; however, in most incidents responders err on the side of transporting too early—a mistake that results in inefficient use of available personnel.

Transportation must not begin until there are enough EMTs on the field to fill all necessary jobs there. As more arrive, the ambulances will begin to travel. For all 10 ambulances to be carrying patients to the hospital, there must be a surplus of at least 10 EMTs over what is needed on the field—i.e., one for each ambulance. Do not, however, wait for all 10 of these extra responders to arrive before beginning transport. Transport can start the minute the first extra responder arrives, and can continue as more responders reach the scene.

As was mentioned earlier, a crew member from each ambulance should always travel in the patient compartment of that ambulance, because he or she will be familiar with the vehicle and its contents in case any supplies are needed en route to the hospital. The driver, however, can be from any crew, or can be a firefighter, or any available responder who has been trained as an emergency vehicle operator.

As more patients and ambulances are ready to leave for the hospital, additional firefighters are needed to help carry and load victims into the ambulances. Firefighters from distant locations should be arriving by now to fill this need. If more are required, take firefighters off the job of transporting victims from the bus to the collecting station, and set them to loading ambulances.

One exceptional possibility bears mention here. At a given point, EMS responders may outnumber the patients. Should this occur, Control may wish to re-evaluate distribution of personnel. It is possible to reassign EMTs so that there is at least one EMT for each patient, no matter where that patient is on the field or what stage of treatment and packaging he has reached. The EMTs would then stay with their patients and move with them throughout the rest of the process, to gain better continuity of care.

BREAKDOWN OF NUMBERS OF RESPONDERS REQUIRED

Three EMTs will fill the command position.
At least 6 will be needed on the bus.
Eight to 10 will be needed to carry victims.
Eight will be needed at the collecting station.
Ten will be needed to drive ambulances.
Ten will be needed in ambulance patient compartments.

The total number of responders required is 45 to 47. This number of responders can handle the 80 to 100 patients that may result from an MCI. Personnel are distributed in sequence as they arrive. This general pattern can always be followed in a closed incident.

Satellite Locations

In certain situations, such as the MGM Grand fire, there will be large numbers of patients suffering from smoke inhalation. Those smoke-inhalation victims who are not otherwise injured can be taken to locations such as a civic center or school gymnasium, instead of to hospitals. At these satellite locations, EMS personnel and laboratory teams can take blood samples to determine which victims could be discharged and which would benefit from hospitalization. Satellite locations, staffed with medical personnel if possible, can be useful in a variety of situations. For example, those who were involved in the incident but who were "unhurt" should be examined. Use of a satellite location for this purpose will cut down on the number of patients being dealt with at the hospitals, freeing hospital staff for the more seriously injured.

Open Incidents

In an open incident, personnel are deployed in a slightly different manner. Since patients are spread over a wide area, it is necessary to locate them before the primary survival scan can commence.

The most efficient way to find the victims is for Control (or Acting Control) to assign incoming responders, in pairs, to search the field. Control should mentally divide the area into 4 or more sectors for searching. As responders arrive, they are paired and sent to the outer perimeter of a sector. Their instructions are to work toward the center of the area, locating and doing primary survival scan on everyone within their sector. Once the primary scan is done on all victims and kraft tags have been applied, each pair of responders goes over its sector again, to assess, stabilize, and package each victim.

In a closed incident, all categories of patients will be brought to the collecting station in mixed order, as they are ready to be taken off the bus. In an open incident, because responders first locate and package the Red patients, Reds will usually reach the collecting station first—with the exception of a few Yellows and Yellow Primes who were stabilized and moved in order to reach some Reds.

When 10 to 12 responders have reached the field and are assessing and packaging patients, the process of carrying patients to the collecting station can begin. Remember, there should be 3 firemen and 1 EMT to carry each patient, and the latter should be the EMT who did the assessment.

In an open incident, Control must balance the number of responders who are out in the field assessing and stabilizing patients with the number who are at the collecting station giving treatment. Where the most responders will be needed will vary from one time in the incident to another.

As soon as enough responders have arrived to continue stabilization and collection of patients and to provide care at the collecting station, the next incoming responders can be used to transport patients to the hospitals.

Aside from the few differences mentioned, deployment of personnel in an open incident is the same as for a closed incident.

Shifting to Hospitals

As the field is cleared of victims, fewer responders are needed in the field—perhaps 4 to 5 to help with victims who may still be trapped, and 2 to 3 ambulances to carry the last victims to hospitals. At this stage, all other EMTs should go to the near hospitals to help treat patients there.

One EMS executive should serve as EMS commander at each hospital. All EMTs at a given hospital will stay with their commander so the hospital staff can locate EMTs for assignments. After completing the assignment, the EMTs will return to their commander for reassignment. In this way, confusion at the hospital will be minimized.

Control will stay in touch with the EMS executive at each hospital to balance the distribution of EMTs, preventing a shortage of help from developing at one hospital when there is a surplus at another.

Utilization of Physicians and Nurses

Primary care physicians, who see patients daily (especially surgeons, Emergency Room physicians, and others accustomed to emergency care), are the ultimate ALS personnel. Their knowledge and expertise make them the very best responders to treat victims of an MCI.

Unfortunately, owing to their medical seniority, physicians are often placed in administrative roles at a Mass Casualty Incident. There are several reasons why this is inadvisable.

1. At any MCI there is such a shortage of medical skills in the field that all physicians should be used to treat patients. (Many senior EMTs can administrate as well as a physician, but EMTs cannot provide medical care at the physician's level.)
2. In few regions do the physicians know the responders well enough to call them by name. They are not used to working with EMTs, firefighters, and police on a daily basis; thus they cannot provide the quality of command that EMS executives can.

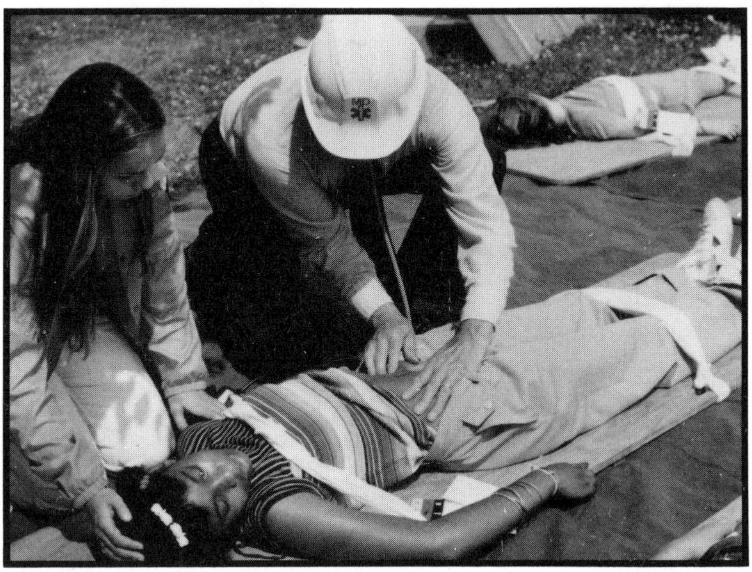

3. Few physicians are experienced in mass casualty response, and few are willing to become involved in the necessary training and drilling. (Ideally, it should be part of the community's mass casualty training program to provide all physicians with at least a minimum of instruction in MCI procedures.)

In the rare event that a physician is available in the field who has had military training in triage (for instance, one who has served in Korea or Viet Nam) he, operating with the Triage Officer, can improve salvage rates. It must be understood, however, that the Triage Officer is still in administrative control. Any other physician or nurse who appears at the site can be invaluable at the collecting station, but should not attempt to administrate site activities.

Though they are not in charge administratively, physicians' decisions should not be challenged on a patient-by-patient basis. However, to avoid counterproductive activity, physicians should be instructed to inform the Triage Officer when they find a patient who should be upgraded. The Triage Officer will then give orders to have that patient moved. Medical personnel should never grab loading personnel and say, "Take this one next." Since the Triage Officer evaluates all of the Red patients, he knows who is most urgently in need of transport. Good communication between medical personnel and the Triage Officer represents the most effective way of dealing with patient priorities.

If IV-qualified nurses arrive on the scene, they should make their presence known. Then, under orders of the Triage Officer or physicians on the field, they should begin administering IVs as indicated. If an IV nurse is not in uniform, he or she can be made instantly identifiable by a simple device: wrap a roller bandage around one arm and write "IV" on it with magic marker.

At the collecting station, after the physicians have treated all Red patients, they should go on to those in the Yellow Prime category. It has been found that more careful diagnosis of Yellow Prime patients will generally locate several who have a better salvage possibility than was first assumed. These patients should be reclassified and transported on a more urgent basis. Where this step has been possible, salvage rates have been increased even beyond the rate inherent in the use of this plan.

Another procedure that should be firmly established on the field is that any nurse or physician who does not know what to do next should report to the Triage Officer, not to Control. Control is in charge of all EMS at the scene. The Triage Officer is responsible for patient care at the collecting station—which should include physicians' and nurses' activities.

It often happens that nurses and physicians from other areas, hearing of the MCI, arrive to offer help. As the field is cleared and there is less for them to do, they may think it is time for them to return home. However, these doctors and nurses can be of help at the near hospitals. Have them check with Control to find out which hospitals can use their assistance before they leave the field.

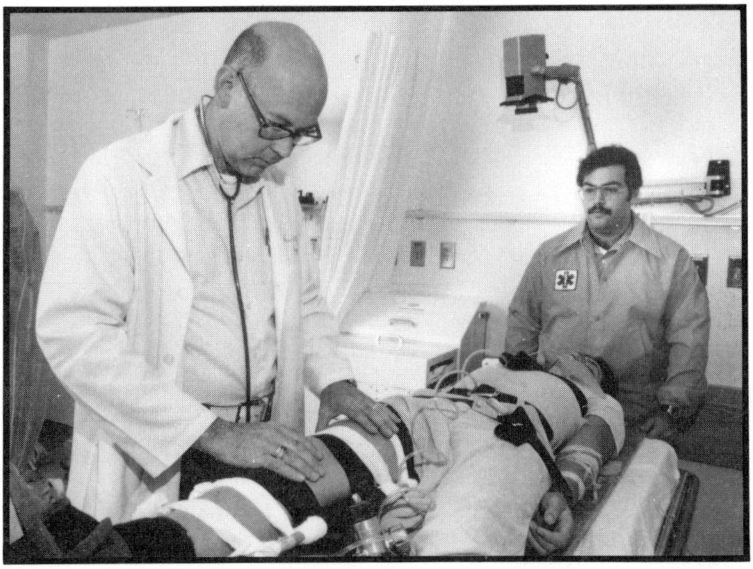

The names and addresses of any doctors and nurses who are involved in rescue and treatment of patients at an MCI should be recorded; these people should be part of the debriefing process and the psychological follow-up discussed in Chapter 12. Nonlocal medical personnel who stopped to help should be apprised of these meetings and urged to attend, to ease the post-incident letdown that can be so debilitating.

Chapter 11
HOSPITAL MCI DISASTER PLANS

Near Hospitals and Far Hospitals

Every hospital must have plans for a variety of contingencies. Guidelines are needed for inhospital fire or bomb threat, strikes by employees, epidemics, and so on. Generally, these plans are functional and realistic. Few hospitals, however, have effective protocols for receiving and handling 25 to 50 patients from a Mass Casualty Incident. Since the specific details of an MCI plan involve such variables as staffing, physical layout, management structure, etc., this chapter will deal with basic concepts and considerations only.

In the event of an MCI, a hospital will either function as a *near* (primary receiving) hospital or a *far* (secondary) hospital. A far hospital receives patients transshipped from a near hospital after they have had some assessment and stabilization, or patients classified Green. This procedure, unfortunately, is alien to most hospitals. In normal practice, the Emergency Department sends people requiring definitive treatment to its own upstairs wards. In a mass casualty situation, the Emergency Department must perceive itself as a stabilization and medical triage center for one to 3 outlying hospitals as well.

The filling and temporary closing down of a near hospital ("Smithfield Hospital to Diaster Control. Don't send us any more patients until further notice.") will result in mistriage. Many patients will have to travel to an outlying hospital an hour or so from the site with no more than rapid field assessment.

This practice will inevitably increase mortality and morbidity. A better method of patient distribution and division of labor is necessary. Although every area and incident will be different, the following guidelines can be adapted to most situations.

Generally there will be one or 2 hospitals within 15 to 25 minutes' running time from the site. The size and capability of these near hospitals is not as important as their ability to receive, evaluate, and stabilize the patients from the site.

Further out will be other hospitals, perhaps 40 to 60 minutes' running time from the site. One of these far hospitals may even be a major medical center.

When an MCI occurs, the ambulances closest to the disaster will move to the site. This leaves the areas normally covered by those ambulances uncovered. To remedy this situation, those ambulances based just outside the area called to the MCI cover the responder's area as well as their own.

The role of the ambulances at the site is to transport patients to the *near* hospital. If there is more than one near hospital, then each should receive roughly the same number of patients (assuming equal stabilization abilities).

Because of pressures at the site and time delays before patients are seen at a medical facility, *all* patients should be transported to a near hospital. The near hospitals should not be bypassed even to transport patients to far hospitals that offer special needed services.

If patients must be transported to a far hospital—either because of the number of patients involved, or because of the in-

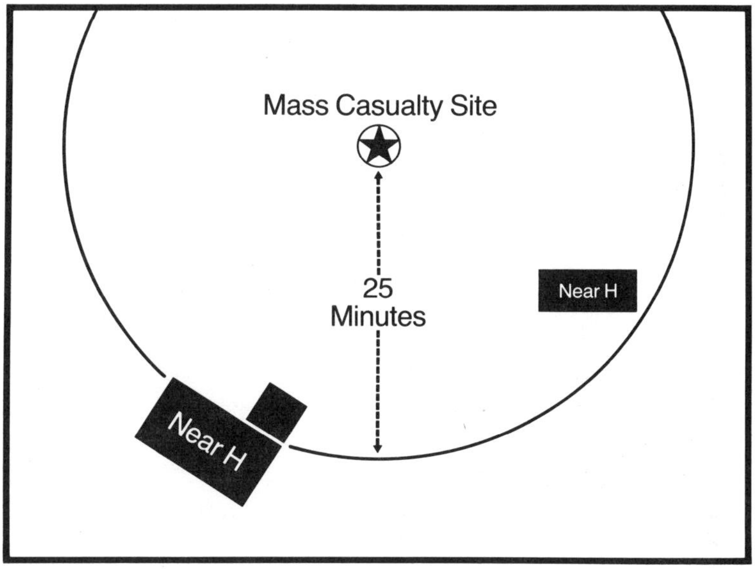

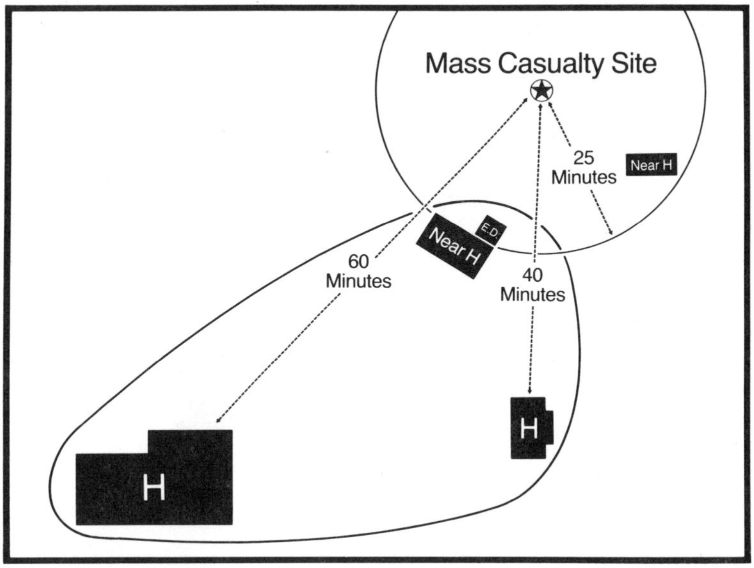

ability of the near hospital to treat certain patients effectively—another approach should be used. The near hospital Emergency Department should notify the far hospital of the situation. Then, it should act as a retriage center and transfer selected patients to the outlying hospitals.

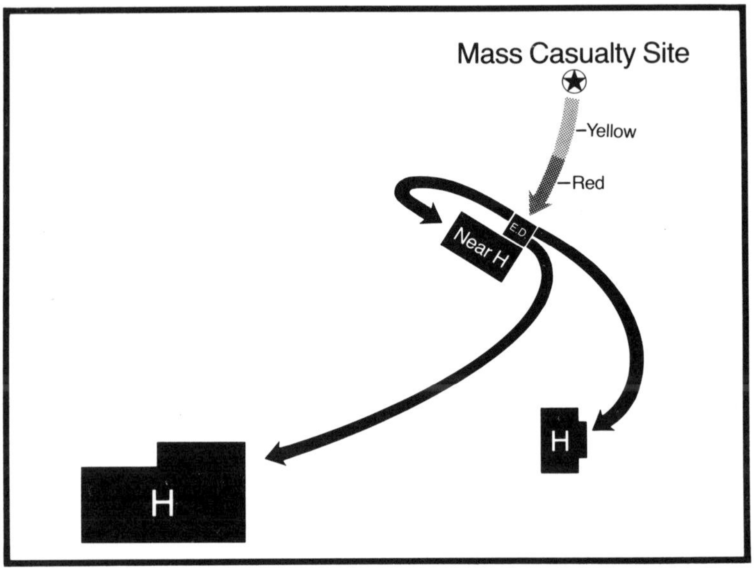

This transfer should not involve the ambulances that respond to the site. Rather, the outlying hospitals should dispatch the ambulances that normally service them to the near hospital. This will

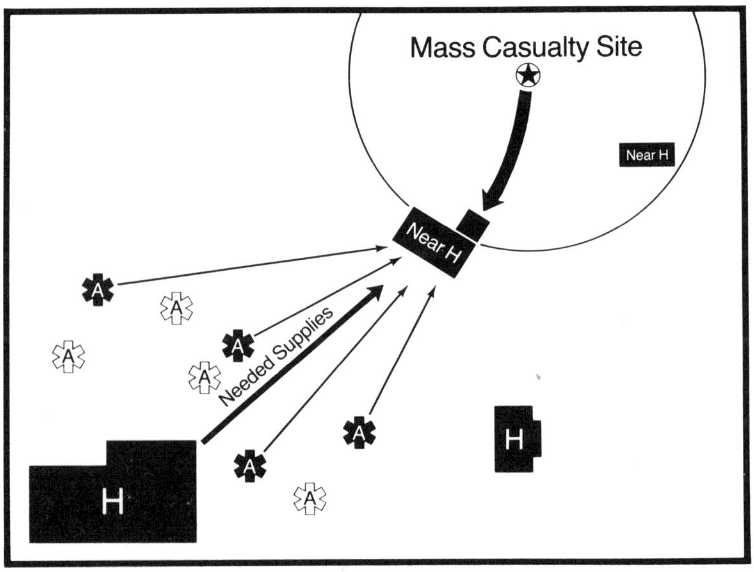

ensure that ambulances continue in a chain between the site and the near hospital, while a separate chain transports designated patients to outlying hospitals.

The field Triage Officer deals with priorities of stabilization and patient removal to the near hospitals. The field Transport Officer establishes an orderly flow to these hospitals and communicates with them. Each near Emergency Department director, often faced with no more than half of the patients from the field, stabilizes, reevaluates, and retriages. He deals with 2 to 3 hospitals, including his own, as treatment facilities. Transporting patients from near to outlying hospitals employs different personnel and vehicles from those responding to the site. This system of compartmentalization places realistic tasks on the field, the near hospitals, and the far hospitals. Each must deal *only* with problems that surround one location.

This system forces re-evaluation, further stabilization, and retriage away from the field into the more favorable environment of a full medical facility. Patients are rechecked, given rapid stabilization treatment as necessary, and transferred to other hospitals. This system also minimizes travel times between evaluations for all patients, not just the "first in." It improves care at every level by spreading the load and reducing tasks to realistic levels.

Only patients with minor injuries, categorized as Green, should be sent directly to outlying hospitals (if the near hospitals cannot handle them). This should be done only after notifying and obtaining the concurrence of the physician in charge of the far hospital's Emergency Department.

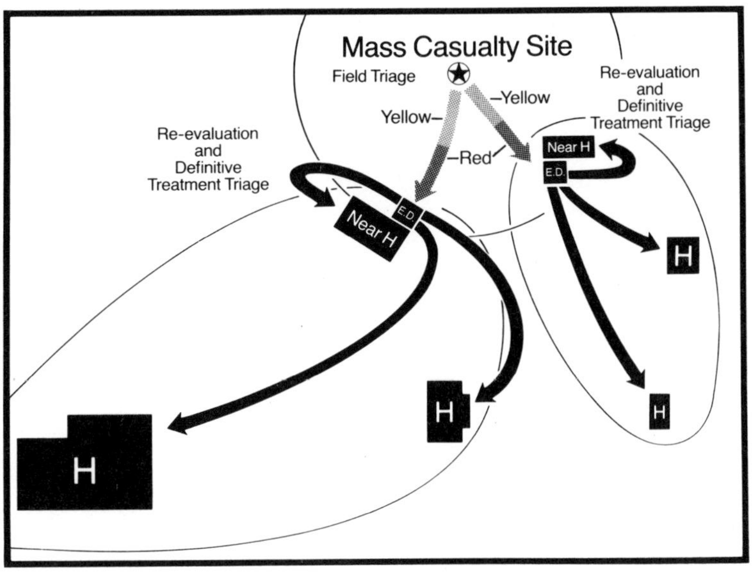

GUIDELINES FOR THE EMERGENCY DEPARTMENT

It is important to remember that field triage is no longer valid at the hospital (except perhaps the distinction between Red and Green patients, who may arrive intermixed). Assessment and distribution of incoming patients is the major initial problem that a good MCI plan must address. Upstaffing floor, laboratory, X-ray, Operating Room, and central materials personnel is difficult but not atypical of other peak upstaffing needs. However, few hospitals have enough room in the Emergency Department to receive, triage, and treat a massive influx of patients. This situation is exacerbated by a loss of working space. Most full service Emergency Departments can handle between 10 and 25 patients at a time (depending on space and staff). It is, however, unlikely that they could cope with an equal number of Reds and Yellow Primes.

The physical separation of the initial receiving area from the Emergency Department is much to be desired—it may even be essential. A large area adjacent to the Emergency Department should be selected. This area should be staffed by a senior, or several, Emergency Department physicians and a senior surgeon.

It is important to take time to re-sort patients, using additional criteria, as soon as they reach the initial receiving area. Remember, most patients will arrive at the hospital in the midst of other patients of approximately the same urgency, based upon field triage. If more than one near hospital exists, the urgent patient load in each will be no more than half the load in the field. Further, these patients will *not* arrive at one time. If a proper rotation system is used among near hospitals, there will be time gaps between incoming ambulances. Even with a lone hospital, gaps will occur.

HOSPITAL ASSESSMENT AND TRIAGE

Several tasks are easily distinguishable for incoming patients. Each patient must be assessed and triaged. If the patient is unstable (therefore, *urgent*) it must be decided whether the patient can be stabilized in the Emergency Department or requires surgical intervention. Since some incoming patients from the disaster and from other sources (regular emergency patients continue to arrive at the hospital) will be fully stable, they may need only interim attention.

In the receiving area each patient is rapidly assessed for 2 considerations:

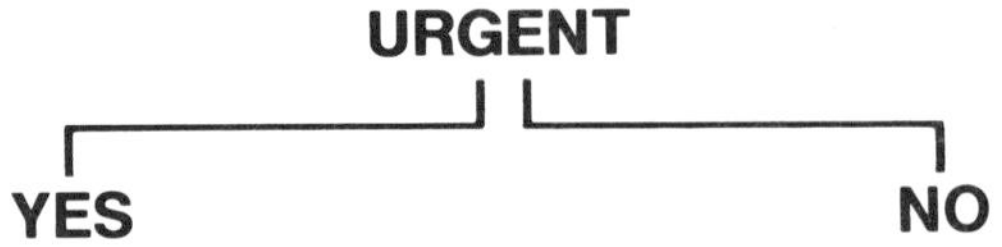

If the evaluation is *no*, the patient should be moved to a holding area and monitored.

The next step is to differentiate the *no*'s. Two types of patients have *no immediate urgent need*. First, there are those with simple injuries that do not commonly have systemic implications. Although these patients may not need definitive medical attention, they may require EMS-provider attention. These patients should be moved to a cafeteria, auditorium, or conference area designated for this purpose. Here, EMTs can monitor them and provide care such as splinting, bandaging, etc.

The second group of patients who may elicit a *no immediate urgent need* response are those whose injuries may eventually produce systemic decline, but who are presently compensating well. Such patients can wait 20 to 40 minutes without any care beyond monitoring and the starting of IV fluids. The designation of a large hallway as an area for holding such patients (in rows on each side of the hall) works well. This area is staffed by IV teams and a physician who is in charge of treatment and patient monitoring.

Patients are continuously monitored at both of these locations; anyone who deteriorates is retriaged as *Urgent*.

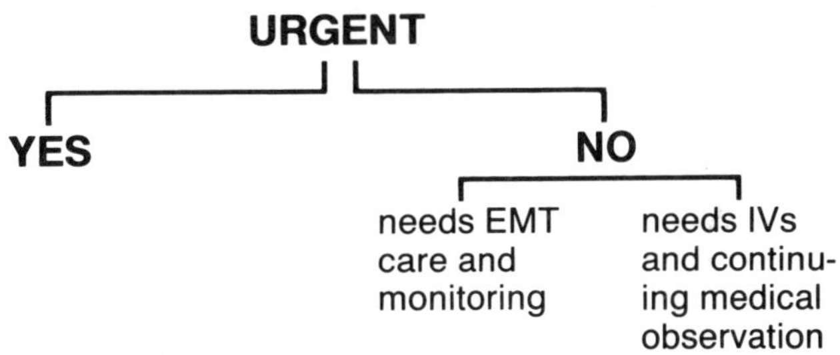

If field triage is proper, most patients who arrive shortly after the disaster will be *urgent—needs immediate attention*. Once the physician in charge of triage at the initial reception area determines that a patient has immediate need for treatment, he must decide whether or not the patient can be stabilized in the Emergency Department. If there is a question, the decision is jointly determined by the Emergency Department physician and the surgeon. If the patient can be stabilized in the Emergency Department, the patient (and his chart) are moved there. If the decision is that surgical intervention is necessary, the senior surgeon, who is in constant touch with an Operating Room management team, assigns the patient to surgery. The patient is then moved up to a preop holding area which is set up for stabilization, examination, and testing.

The chief of surgery, or his senior delegate, reviews patients holding for surgery and, on the basis of urgency, available instruments, and salvageability, selects the next case as each

Operating Room becomes available. Selection must also consider one other factor. While more patients are still arriving, or are immediately expected, all Operating Rooms should not simultaneously become involved in what are estimated to be long procedures. If possible, attempt selection so that at least one Operating Room becomes free every 30 minutes or so to accommodate an arriving patient who is eminently salvageable if treated quickly.

The scope of the incident and the expected number of patients will determine the degree of immediate surgical repair beyond that necessary for stabilization. It is important that ORs not be blocked by a great deal of "total patient repair." For example, it would be inadvisable to undertake reduction of extremity fractures that do not involve neurological or circulatory impairment while other patients needing intrathoracic or intra-abdominal intervention are waiting. Stabilization and intervention must be the prime consideration, even if it will necessitate a second scheduling for additional surgical repair.

Some of the patients stabilized in the Emergency Department will not need surgery at all, or at least not for several hours. These patients are admitted and moved upstairs for floor care. Others, however, even though presently stable, will need surgery in the next several hours. Based upon an evaluation of the "most urgent" surgical load, a case-by-case decision whether to hold or transship these patients will have to be made.

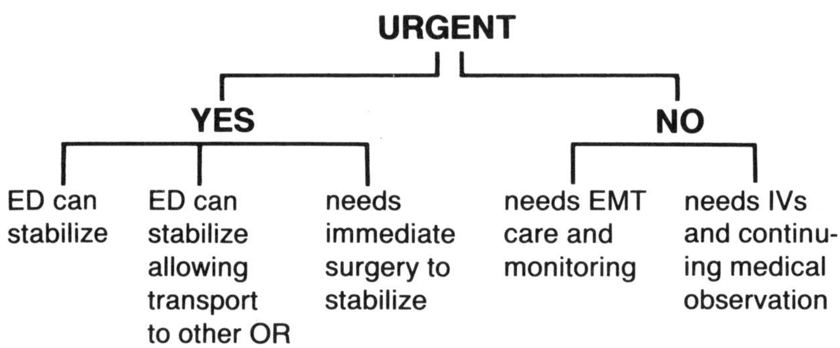

Although experience shows hospitals are instinctively loath to transship, this is a better, safer system than shipping patients from the field to far hospitals. The leapfrogging of urgent trauma patients past near hospitals to outlying facilities involves lengthy transport times and contributes to mortality in 2 ways: directly, to those patients who are so transported without reassessment and retriage; and indirectly, to those still awaiting transportation, since the extensive travel times will reduce the availability of ambulances in the field.

Chapter 12
THE PSYCHOLOGICAL AFTERMATH

Psychological Impact of an MCI

A Mass Casualty Incident may produce a scene of carnage so devastating that no description can adequately convey what it was like to be involved. The pain and horror—the feelings of fear and despair, of tension and urgency and rage; the sight of so many dismembered or disemboweled victims, of blood and brains and intestines splattered about; the sound of people in agony screaming for help; the indescribable smell of blood and death—normal human experience does not include any of this. Even day-to-day EMS duties do not involve these experiences in the hellish quantity an MCI can produce.

No one—*no one*—be he responder, victim, or witness, can walk away from such a nightmare untouched.

A Mass Casualty Incident changes the lives of the people involved—sometimes seriously, sometimes permanently. For varying periods of time afterward, everyone who was present will be in some stage of mental and/or emotional crisis. Most of them will need help. The mass casualty response plan should take into consideration this very real need, and include plans to deal with it.

It is important to understand at the outset that people can be in emotional or mental crisis *without being mentally ill*. There should be no stigma attached to the fact that the victims of a mass casualty—and emotionally, the responders as well as the patients are victims—may need some form of professional counseling to help them cope with the trauma they have been through.

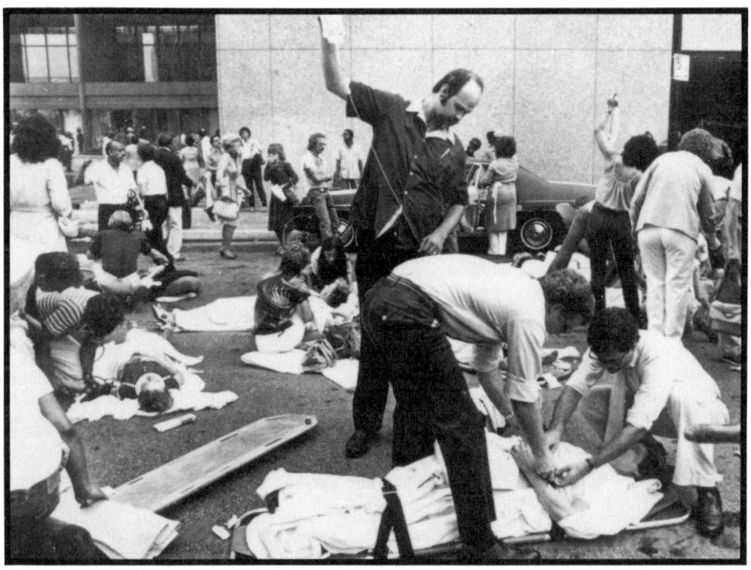

United Press International Photo

Causes and Effects of Emotional Trauma

People who have not responded to an MCI sometimes find it hard to comprehend why the participants may take weeks or months to "snap out of it." It may be helpful, therefore, to understand what it is about a Mass Casualty Incident that causes so much emotional distress, and what the results can be.

Three groups are considered *at risk* after an MCI: responders, survivors, and relatives.

Responders. By responders we mean all fire, police, and emergency medical personnel at the scene; all of the involved personnel at the near hospital, including doctors, and nurses; and any other hospital personnel at farther hospitals who may have had to deal with possibly overwhelming numbers of victims. All of these individuals are included, regardless of the length of time they were involved. The last ambulance crew to arrive is just as much at risk as the first.

It is important to remember that this definition of *responder* includes those doctors who where involved in treating the victims. Many people—including doctors themselves—feel that the doctors are inured to the sight of maimed and broken bodies. This may be true on an individual-patient basis. But nothing in everyday medical practice, nor even in everyday Emergency Room practice, could prepare a doctor for the sight of 20 or 30 badly injured patients *whom he does not have time or facilities to treat as completely as his training and knowledge would normally permit*. The decisions he will have to make and the tensions he will undergo, are *not* within his normal experience; and, therefore, he may be even more at risk mentally and emotionally than other responders.

Following are some negative feelings commonly produced by an MCI.

1. *Feeling of inadequacy*. Even the most dedicated, well-trained responder is likely to be completely overwhelmed by the sight of so much human tragedy. He will almost certainly be so upset that for the first few minutes he will be unable to function as efficiently as he himself expected. And after he pulls himself together and sets to work, he may still find himself distracted, unable to perform as well as he can with individual patients on a normal basis. He will feel inadequate.

2. *Feelings of frustration and powerlessness*. The responder will be forced to bypass victims that, under other circumstances, he would make every effort to save. Even though he knows that passing over those with low salvageability increases the total survival rate, he will feel frustrated and powerless at his inability to help everyone.

3. *Fear*. Often there is an element of physical danger at the scene of a Mass Casualty Incident. Will the suspended bus go over the edge of the bridge? Will the gas tank explode before everyone can be taken to safety? Responders working under this kind of pressure suffer from fear for their own safety.

Responders may also suffer from *fear of making a mistake*. Lives are in the balance; a wrong decision can mean an unnecessary death. Triage Officers are particularly susceptible to this fear, since making God-like decisions is the purpose of their job.

4. *Guilt*. Responders are also likely to suffer from feelings of guilt: guilt over real or imagined misjudgments; guilt over casual handling of the dead or moribund; guilt over "playing God." Responders who were unable to hold up throughout the entire incident will feel guilty over "letting everyone down."

5. *Insecurity*. Having witnessed this example of the inscrutability of fate, a responder may later begin to feel a lack of faith in life's rationality. If 30 people can be killed at home in their beds by an apartment fire, then where are you safe? What can you depend on? The responder may begin to have feelings of insecurity.

Any or all of these feelings—inadequacy, frustration, powerlessness, fear, guilt, and insecurity—can build up in a responder during and after the incident. If not dealt with, they can have serious consequences for the individual's mental stability.

He may begin to doubt his competence to deal with life's daily matters. (Maybe he shouldn't try to insulate the attic himself—it might be better to call in a professional who'll be sure to do it right.) Suddenly he is unable to make up his mind about the simplest matters. (Should he wash the car today, or should he mow the lawn instead? Making the choice seems to be too much for him, so he may do neither.)

He may become nervous, tense, and irritable. When problems arise, he may yell at people instead of trying to work things out calmly. Or he may withdraw from his family and friends—become moody and depressed, forgetful.

Virtually every responder will suffer some of these reactions to some degree. Some people may be able to pull themselves out within a few days, with the support of family and friends. Others, however, may need special help. Everyone has different threshholds of tolerance for this type of mental stress; it is no reflection on an EMT's abilities if he finds himself unable to recover from an MCI without some form of assistance.

Survivors. This includes all victims who survived the crash, whether they were injured or not. In some cases, those who survive without injury are more in need of counseling than those who are seriously injured.

Survivors of an MCI are affected by some factors that are different from those affecting responders.

1. *Emotional shock of impact*. Imagine a 40-year-old woman who boards a bus with her 10-year-old daughter and her 7-year-old son for a sightseeing tour in the mountains. They are debating whether to call Dad at lunchtime or at dinner, when suddenly, with no warning, the bus goes off the road and rolls down the mountainside. Thirty seconds later, the woman is badly injured, her daughter is dead, she can't find her son at all, and there are unimaginable sights and sounds all around her. Nothing in her life will ever be the same again—and it all happened in one unbelievable half-minute. This woman and all the other survivors of the accident will be affected by the emotional shock of impact.

2. *Helplessness and isolation*. The victim described above will be taken out of the bus and cared for by helpful strangers who will probably be unable to tell her anything about her son or daughter. She will be taken to a strange hospital where she will be cared for kindly, but quickly and impersonally—there are so many others needing care. She will feel helpless and isolated without her loved ones.

3. *Survival guilt*. She will be distraught over her daughter's death and her son's disappearance. They are dead, while she is still alive. She will feel guilty for having survived. (This particular reaction may be more severe if the survivor is uninjured or not seriously hurt. Survival guilt can occur even if the survivor did not know any of the other victims in the accident. To be alive when others are dead may seem to some people an undeserved reward.)

4. *Blaming*. Children and even adults may blame the entire accident on themselves: "I'm being punished because I once *wished* my Mom was dead." This blaming creates more guilt in the survivor's mind.

5. *Anxiety*. Of course, if she is injured, the survivor will be worried about herself as well. Will she be disfigured? Disabled? Will she be able to afford all the treatment she will need? She will be filled with anxiety for a variety of reasons.

All of these factors and feelings—shock of impact, helplessness, isolation, survival guilt, blaming, and anxiety—can build up over a period of days or weeks. If they are not recognized and dealt with, they can have a lasting effect on the survivor and her family.

Survivors of an MCI may also suffer from the feeling that life has lost its meaning and rationality, that it has become "unreal." They may become depressed, feeling that there's "no point in trying to go on."

Survivors may suffer from nervousness and be afraid to let their loved ones out of their sight. The subconscious thought here is, "What if it happens again?"

They may also be bothered by recurring, unbidden memories of the event—a certain sound or smell may trigger visual images of the accident, bringing everything back to them over and over again. These recurring flashbacks, which can be so abrupt and unexpected as to cause startle reactions, are very stressful.

Like the responders, survivors may become anxious, moody, and forgetful, unable to make decisions. They may flare up easily over small problems.

Relatives. This includes relatives of survivors and relatives of those who died. It also includes survivors who lost relatives in the incident.

1. *Uncertainty*. Relatives may suffer stress from prolonged periods of uncertainty as to the fate of their family members.
2. *Emotional shock of impact*. Like the survivors, they are affected by the emotional shock of impact; in a moment, their lives are changed through no act of their own.
3. *Blaming*. They may, nonetheless, blame themselves, just as the survivors do.
4. *Survival guilt.*
5. *Separation anxiety.* They may go through separation anxiety: "Last time she went away, she was nearly killed. I'm not letting her out of my sight!"

Relatives may suffer from many of the same symptoms the survivors do. Relatives of dead or severely injured victims may go through a period of over-activity, of frenetic attempts to cope. When this period of activity ends (for instance, when the funeral is over, or when the fate of the loved one seems certain) the relative may lapse into deep depression and inactivity.

Providing Psychological Assistance

It should be part of the response plan to provide counseling for everyone involved in a Mass Casualty Incident.

Responders. For responders, psychological help in coping with the stress of an MCI can begin before the incident occurs. Mass casualty training sessions should include pretraining in the mental and emotional effects to be anticipated. This training should be conducted by a group of competent mental health professionals, who will then remain involved in the community's total response plan.

This pretraining should make several things clear:

1. Everyone should expect to be affected in some way by a Mass Casualty Incident. To show signs of stress during and after

the incident is entirely normal and is in no way to be taken as a sign of weakness. Anyone who thinks, "Well, I'm tough; I can take it; it won't get to me," is setting himself up for trouble.

2. It sometimes happens that a responder becomes so overwhelmed by the magnitude of an MCI, and by the conditions under which he must function, that his performance is affected. When this happens, the responder must be able to admit that he is not coping, and that he must withdraw from the scene. This is not "copping out"; this is mature, responsible behavior. All responders must be trained in "self-withdrawal analysis"—so that they will recognize when they have reached the point of dysfunction. Should this occur, they will understand that for the security of the scene, as well as for their own mental and emotional stability, they must stop attempting to treat victims, and report to Control that they are withdrawing.

3. It must be understood by everyone that if a responder feels it necessary to withdraw, this does not mean that he is not an effective EMT. He will probably still be able to function effectively in daily EMS situations and should not feel obligated to retire from the team.

Pretraining should include a visit from someone who has been through an MCI—possibly someone from another area. This speaker should describe the scene of the incident he witnessed as graphically as possible, not in medical terms, but in terms of human tragedy and destruction. This is the closest your team is likely to come to a preunderstanding of what the scene will be like without actually going through an incident, and it will be helpful in preparing team members for what they are likely to see and hear.

The counselors conducting these pretraining sessions may be psychologists or lay social workers. Ideally, they should be trained in emergency medicine, so there will be some common bond of understanding between them and the responders. If this is not possible, try to provide the counselors with some experience in EMS—riding the ambulance for a week, perhaps, or attending classes or lectures.

It is important that the counselors, from then on, be considered part of the response plan. Thus, after an incident, the responders will be dealing with counselors who are already familiar to them. This will minimize any initial awkwardness involved in discussing intense, potentially embarrassing feelings with strangers.

It should be noted that the group of counselors can be expanded to include members of the clergy if this would be of support to any of the responders.

As soon as possible after the incident is over, and certainly within 24 hours, there should be a debriefing session for all responders—police, fire, and EMS personnel—as well as hospital personnel, including doctors and nurses. These sessions, though they should be led by members of the group of counselors, should be relatively unstructured. A guest psychologist who is experienced in emotional reactions to an MCI, might be invited to deliver a talk on the effects of an MCI on responders; however, the main purpose of these sessions is to allow the responders to talk out their feelings.

At these sessions, responders should be encouraged to discuss any feelings of failure or insecurity they may have felt, and to tell of any particularly painful incidents that happened to them—to talk about the woman who cried for help, but had to be passed over because she had no chance to survive; or the dismembered child; or the patient who died just as the rescuers got to him. Responders should also be encouraged to describe any feelings of pride at having been able to help or save someone.

It should not be expected that any conclusions will be reached at these sessions. In fact, these discussions must not be permitted to involve any considerations of whose fault it was that things went wrong, or how things might have been done better. These matters can be discussed at another time. The focus of these sessions is to allow the responders to bring to light hidden feelings, to talk about them, and to discover that everyone had the same reactions. The sooner these mutual emotions can be aired, the less chance there is that any individual will suppress his real feelings. Suppressing deep emotions doesn't make them go away; they will only crop up in disguise later on, and be more difficult to deal with.

These meetings should be very valuable to responders. However, intervention should not stop here. All responders should be required to meet with one of the mental health counselors several times over the next 6 months. In addition, the plan should include the option, for each responder, of having continuing, private meetings with a counselor, for as long as it is necessary to help the responder feel secure again.

It should be emphasized that Triage Officers, by the nature of their role, are placed under unimaginable mental and emotional stress during an incident. Theirs is the judgment that lets one man die untreated so that another man may be treated and live. And this choice must be made not once, but many times during an MCI. The emotional and mental repercussions of these decisions can be traumatic in the extreme. Therefore, the Triage Officer should be offered intensive, in-depth therapy for as long as necessary.

Families of responders. The counselors should make contact with the families of the responders, explain what the responder has been through and is now going through, tell them what signs of stress to watch for, and offer help to family members who need support as a result of problems caused by the responder's reaction to the MCI. A son, for instance, may feel neglected because his father can't seem to get interested in playing baseball with him any more; or a husband may be distressed at his wife's lack of interest in sex since she responded to the MCI.

Family members, and the responders themselves, should watch in particular for any signs that emotions about the incident are being masked. Denial of stress can in itself be a sign of stress, and as has been pointed out, when emotions are suppressed they may simply resurface later in other ways.

Counseling should be available to all responders without charge. The EMS, fire, police, and hospital personnel who responded to the MCI, whether paid or volunteer, have performed a service for the community that goes beyond the normal definition of duty. They do it because it has to be done and they have the ability to do it. They want to do it, to help people who are in need. If the responders are then themselves in need of help, no responsible community will withhold treatment of what must be considered a job-related injury. The town should automatically take care of any bills submitted for counseling related to an MCI.

Assistance for Survivors in the Community

Perhaps the most devastating type of Mass Casualty Incident is that which involves only or mainly members of one community—a school bus accident, for example, or the collapse of bleachers at a local football game. This type of incident, in which victims and responders know or are even related to each other, is more traumatic for everyone—survivors and responders alike—than any other kind. Indeed, an MCI of this nature places stress on the entire community, and calls for a special effort to help restore everyone's mental balance.

If it is found that a member of any responder's family is a victim of the incident, that family member should be stabilized and transported immediately, accompanied by that responder, regardless of how serious or mild his injury is. Knowledge that responder's families will be given priority provides the maximum peace of mind for all responders and will improve their morale, leading to improved effectiveness. If a responder should become a victim, he too should be transported immediately. This also makes for improved morale on the part of the other responders at the scene.

News about a local disaster always seems to travel fast. Frightened relatives begin showing up at the scene, worried about their loved ones, full of questions, and sometimes interfering with rescue efforts. It is wise to arrange for a school bus to carry relatives to the hospitals so they can locate their family members. In fact, a driver for such a bus should be on the call-up list.

In the hours and days following the incident, a school bus should be detailed to make regular runs from a central location, such as the town hall, to all the local hospitals where victims are being cared for. This will make life easier for the families involved.

If possible, a mental health professional or a member of the clergy should visit the families of all victims of the incident—including the families of those who died. Where this is not feasible, the use of EMS personnel may be considered. During the visit, it should be explained to the relatives that they will surely be undergoing extreme mental and emotional stress. Provide a phone number they can call if they require any kind of help—emotional or practical. Set up a hot line for families of victims, and encourage them to make use of the service.

The community as a whole should be helped to realize that the families involved in the MCI are undergoing stress, and that the behavior of these people may temporarily change as they adjust to their new circumstances.

In the face of the disruption an accident can cause, the normal demands of life may be too much for the families to bear. Some or all of these services may be needed.

1. Babysitting.
2. Transportation around town.
3. Cooking.
4. Housekeeping.
5. Help in making funeral arrangements.
6. Financial support.

There are various local agencies in almost any town that are equipped with resources and contacts to provide these services: the Red Cross, Kiwanis, or VFW, for instance.

Don't expect the families of the victims to call and ask for support. Most of them will not do so. Social agency or EMS personnel may have to call them, or drop by and make concrete, practical offers of assistance: "Don't worry about the laundry, Mrs. Barnes. I can have someone here in 15 minutes to do that for you. You just get on over to the hospital; your husband needs you."

Too often, a community will make supreme efforts to help the families of the victims for a few days . . . and then things will go back to normal. But these people will continue to need help for weeks and months after the crisis has passed. This help should be available to them for as long as they need it.

Community involvement of this nature is not only supportive of the families in need; it is also helpful in the healing process that the entire community must go through to recover from an MCI.

Chapter 13

PREPLANNING, PREPAREDNESS, AND TRAINING

Local Needs and Problems

The plan presented in this book is a generalized one. It comprises an overview of the mass casualty response. In order to have meaning for all responders, it deals with the most common types of incidents in the most typical kinds of terrain.

But no MCI or region is entirely typical. There are always situations and combinations of circumstances that are unique to a given incident or area. Therefore, the plan must be adapted to fit specific needs.

Shaping this general plan into a specific one for any given area involves 3 steps, the first 2 of which occur in the preplanning stage.

1. **Understanding the general plan.** All responders should become familiar with the plan presented in this book. Everyone—executive personnel, ambulance crews, the dispatchers—should understand what an MCI is, how and why a mass casualty response differs from daily EMS care of patients, and how the areas of command should be organized.

Many of the general rules laid out in this book are applicable to any incident anywhere. For instance, there must *always* be a Triage Officer, a Transportation Officer, and a Control Officer. If all responders understand that fact, and know whom to contact with specific problems, there will be less confusion in the field.

However, some aspects of this plan may not be directly applicable to certain areas. Therefore, Step 2 is necessary.

2. **Adapting this general plan into a localized, written plan.** This involves preplanning based upon knowledge of the local people, geography, climate, equipment, and so forth. For instance, getting an ambulance to certain areas of Montana, even in reasonable weather, normally takes 2 hours. Remember that in an MCI, responders will be unable to do better than they do under daily emergency conditions—indeed, the goal is to do no worse. Therefore, the mass casualty response plan for that area must take the 2-hour time factor into consideration. The local EMS must either allow for it in their system, or they must make prior arrangements for helicopters.

Adapting this plan requires meetings with the heads of local government and the other emergency agencies to determine specific needs and problems, and to work out a general methodology that will deal with those needs and problems.

Once the needs and problems have been resolved, a local call-up plan can be established. This plan must be written down, and it must be complete in every detail.

All of the agencies involved—EMS, fire, police, rescue, hospitals, and local government, plus any others specifically required for a given area—must understand their responsibilities during an MCI in *each* town in the region before specific training in local procedures can begin. In other words, the Weston emergency agencies must know what to do for an MCI in Weston, and also what they are to do for an MCI in Easton, Wilton, Danbury, Norwalk, and so on.

It is recommended that all towns in a region go through the same general training program to ensure that everyone is trained in the same system. Each town should also be aware, however, of specific problems in neighboring towns, and of how those problems will be handled. For instance, if one town covers a wilderness area that can only be reached by canoe, all neighboring towns that would be called in for an MCI in that location must know what plans have been made to deal with the situation.

The third step takes place in the event of an incident.

3. **Adapting the town's plan for a specific MCI.** Each incident has its own set of problems and peculiarities, which must be dealt with *as the response is taking place*. One incident may take place in an isolated ravine, necessitating horses and riders to bring equipment and evacuate patients. Another may involve hazardous materials that need special handling. A third may involve victims flung over a wide area, adding to the problems of triage and treatment. The local plan will have to be modified for each incident. Consequently, the person who will make these adaptations must be identified in the plan.

This does not mean that the same individual must take on this responsibility for every MCI in the area; instead, it means that whoever fills a given function—usually Control—will be the one who gives the final orders to deviate from the plan. It is important that the person who is responsible for this function—which requires *aggressive field initiative*—be *on-site*. Any attempt to modify the general plan or control events from a hospital or town hall can only result in delays and inappropriate activity that will have an adverse effect on salvage rates.

A Preplanning and Training Sequence

EMS personnel, in working with police, fire, and rescue representatives to create local response plans, may end up at a disadvantage if they don't clearly understand what they are negotiating for. They often have no clearly established line of command, as do the police and fire departments, and, therefore, have difficulty in establishing their position in the negotiations. It should be established ahead of time who will represent the EMS group, and those individuals must clearly understand their goals and responsibilities in the negotiations. If *all* EMS personnel are trained in the general response plan presented in this book, their understanding of an MCI will be a useful negotiating tool. Therefore, the following outline is suggested in preplanning for an MCI.

1. Train all EMS personnel in the general response considerations that apply to most MCIs—in other words, the overall plan presented in this book. Make sure that each individual understands the *whys* and *wherefores* of every step.

2. Establish the procedures that will be followed by all EMS responders at an MCI. Predetermine who will be the key MCI executive—and have more than one person ready to fill each position in case someone cannot be located in time. Be sure that all EMS responders know who their executives are.

3. Negotiate the local plan with other agencies. Establish procedures that will be followed by fire, police, rescue, civil preparedness, local hospitals, government, etc.

4. Codify a local plan with specific details for all departments and agencies.

5. Train all EMS personnel in that codification. (At the same time, fire, police, rescue, and all other involved agencies should be receiving training in the procedures they are to follow.)

6. EMS executives should run one-hour information sessions for local police, fire, rescue, civil preparedness, and government officials, and for hospital Emergency Department staff. These sessions should brief the other agencies on what the EMS will be doing at an MCI, what the special EMS problems are at an MCI, and particularly how and why triage differs from what is done on daily EMS calls. This step should promote swift understanding and willing cooperation between the EMS and all other agencies.

7. Run a series of EMS practice classes and drills as described in the rest of this chapter.

Practice Classes and Drills

It would be criminally irresponsible to teach a novice how to use a backboard by taking him to the scene of an accident and using victims for demonstration and practice. It is equally irresponsible to teach the skills required at an MCI on the site of an actual disaster. Classroom instruction and drill are necessary to learn these special skills.

Once all regional needs and problems have been resolved; once the call-up procedures are solidified; once all EMTs understand the philosophy behind mass casualty reponse; and once they have learned the general procedures that will be followed in a given area, it is time to begin hands-on practice in the skills and techniques required.

First, all EMTs must be taught triage, rapid assessment, and rapid packaging. *Do not* assume that a knowledge of assessment and packaging for daily EMS application is sufficient. An MCI, with its special time-frame and patient-quantity problems, calls for modifications in both these skills.

When the basic skills have been learned in the classroom, practice drills can begin.

It is a common error for overeager EMS teams to leap from the classroom directly into "real-life" drills with mock patients, real equipment, waiting ambulances, and plenty of enthusiasm. Almost inevitably the trainees forget that this is intended to be a *learning* experience. They begin to role-play. Soon there are scores of EMTs running around attempting to clear the field too fast, getting more and more frantic as it becomes apparent that they haven't enough knowledge and understanding to deal with a mock drill. How will they ever be able to cope with a real disaster?

This mistake—and the depression and sense of futility it engenders—can be avoided by following a sequence of drills designed to familiarize the EMTs with the procedures they will follow at an MCI.

Some areas run one drill a year; some run 2 or 3. However often drills occur, each should increase only one step in complexity, as described below.

1. Begin with one or more card drills in the classroom. Using triage practice cards, have the trainees read the symptoms, determine the probable injuries and status, and place the cards in triage rows on the classroom floor.

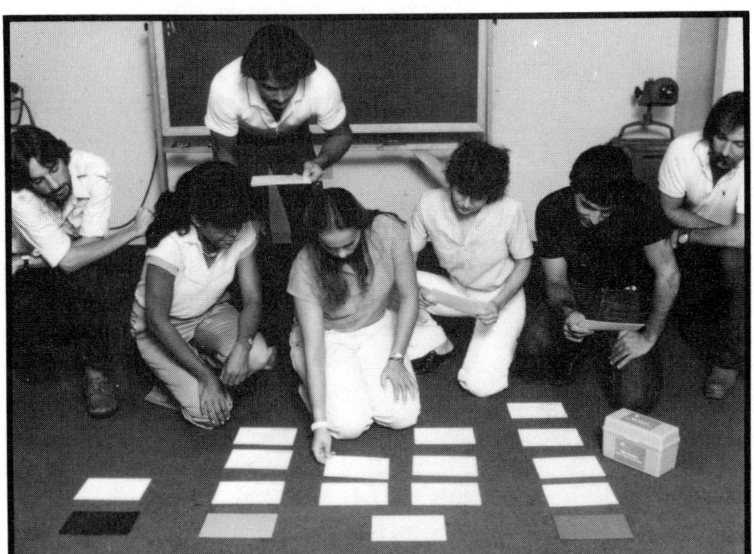

2. Run a "gymnasium" drill. (Any large room will do, but a gymnasium is probably best.) Have mock patients, each with one of the triage cards to describe his "condition." This drill should be conducted slowly and deliberately. There should be no sense of hurry as "patients" are assessed and packaged using the techniques, but not the normal speed, of rapid packaging. Real equipment—backboards, bandages, etc., should be used. In fact, this drill can be considered a "checklist" to see that all equipment is available. The patients should be carried to the triage station. This drill will provide experience in actual manipulation of patients, as well as practice in bandaging and rapid packaging.

3. Run a "dress rehearsal" for EMTs. This drill should be a "slow-motion" walk-through, using mock patients and triage cards as was done in the "gymnasium" drill. The director of this drill should use a public address system to describe to each group what they are to do next.

4. Have a "slow-motion" walk-through for everybody—the EMS, fire, police, rescue, Emergency Room, and whatever other services are included in your local protocols.

5. Now, the community is ready to have that "real-life" drill. Backed by practice in rapid assessment and packaging, EMTs and their fellow responders will be able to get the most out of the situation.

Continue to use triage cards for the first "real-life" drill. Do not use makeup or have the patients act out their complaints. Also, do not attempt a "surprise" drill at this stage. All personnel should know where and when the drill will occur. Choose a simple, easily accessible closed incident, something like the one in Chapter 5. (Open incidents should be practiced separately, later on, since they involve more complexities and difficulties than are found in closed incidents.)

6. For the next "real-life" drill, move to a more remote location, but continue to use the cards to identify each patient's particular condition.

7. For the following drill, notify personnel only that there will be a mock MCI "sometime this month." The exact date and location can be a surprise. For this drill, makeup and acting could be used. In that case, only the patient sees his triage card. As the responder goes through the rapid assessment, the patient gives, at the appropriate moment, his vital statistics. He says, for instance, "You have just felt a fracture of the left femur," as the responder palpates that area. If the responder doesn't ask for the right information, the patient doesn't volunteer it. This approximates what happens when a responder fails to perform all parts of a rapid survey. (Obviously this type of drill requires knowledgeable "patients" who have been thoroughly briefed in their roles.)

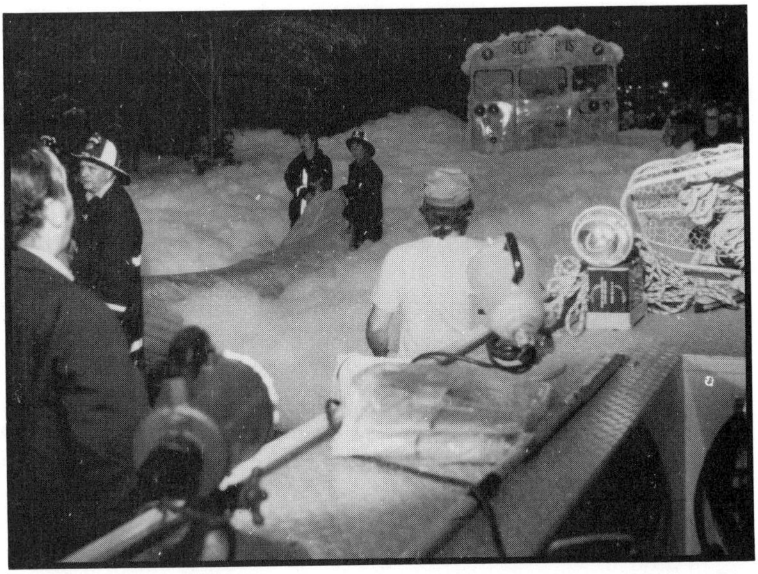

The increments in the complexity of drills are flexible. It may prove advisable to repeat one step or eliminate others, depending upon what is appropriate for the personnel. It may even be possible to proceed to a still more lifelike drill, such as the one recently done in our own area.

We found an unusable school bus, took it out to a deserted stretch of road, and turned it over on its side. On the rear door we put a sign: "Buckled—cannot be used." (We left the door operable, however, for safety's sake.) Thus, entrance had to be effected through the windscreen and by peeling back part of the roof.

"Patients" were placed in the overturned bus. A safe distance away, we placed the "other car" in the "incident," dug a trench around it, and with fire lines in place for safety, ignited this vehicle.

The exercise was run in the evening, with limited light. Rescue personnel had to find entrance and egress. The burning vehicle added an extra element of realism—the smell and sound of the fire, and the excitement of fire-suppression activities, lent urgency to the incident, thus more closely approximating the conditions to be found at a real incident.

Needless to say, if we had tried this complex a drill our first time out, we would probably have ended up caring for some real injuries. However, because we had built up gradually to this drill, everything went smoothly—at least, as smoothly as things are ever likely to go at an MCI!

Drills up to and including the dress rehersal should be completed within 12 months. Ensuing drills may be scheduled 6 months to a year apart.

PRECAUTIONS DURING DRILLS

Mass Casualty Incident drills are an invitation to *real* trouble. Any time you have a large number of people and vehicles involved in activities in a limited area, there is the possibility of real illness or injury. Furthermore (as some EMS groups have discovered) when a large number of local ambulances and personnel are taken out of daily circulation even for a short time, a *true* emergency seems bound to occur—requiring the return of some ambulances and personnel. Therefore, whenever preparing for a drill the following possibilities must be considered.

1. **A real victim at the drill**. At one drill we know of, a fireman suffered a heart attack. The problem was discovered immediately, and the man was taken to the hospital in the next available ambulance. However, there was a failure in communications somewhere along the way. When the fireman arrived at the Emergency Department, he was grouped with the mock patients from the drill. The true nature of his condition was discovered by accident in the course of the hospital's drill procedures. The dangers of this happening are evident. There are 2 possible solutions.
   a. A coded "cancel exercise" signal is transmitted over all frequencies to hospital, fire, police, rescue, etc. Upon receipt of this signal, all drill activities cease until the true emergency has been dealt with. This system minimizes the possibility of miscommunication between the various areas of operation.
   b. A field executive from the drill site, after notifying the hospital that a true emergency has occurred, accompanies the ambulance with the real patient. A few minutes before arriving at the hospital he can reinforce his earlier notification by calling again with a reminder that he will be there in a few minutes. "Park City Hospital, this is Weston Unit 50 with a *real* patient—a 48-year-old heart attack victim; we are 3 minutes from your location."

Throughout the hospital, all drill activities and mock triage should stop until the real patient is stabilized. Only then can the drill resume in the hospital and in the field.

2. **A real emergency call for one of the services taking part in the drill**. In the event of, say, a fire in a town whose engines are taking part in the drill, a prearranged signal should be broadcast from a central dispatcher to indicate that a true emergency is coming in. Everyone on the field should sit quietly so that commands can be heard over the PA system. An on-site executive should then issue commands to clear the necessary areas of the field to permit the safe withdrawal of the vehicles needed for the true emergency.

Other precautionary measures can minimize the danger of real injury and the possible confusion of real patients with mock patients.

1. The triage tags themselves are a safeguard. The mere presence of such a card on a patient during drill tells which patients are mock. However, all personnel involved in triaging on the field should be instructed to write *MOCK* clearly on the triage tag. This would prevent confusion in the not entirely impossible event that a *true Mass Casualty Incident occurred during a drill*. (In this event, of course, the drill ceases immediately and the mock patients should be instructed to leave the hospital. However, there is no harm in taking that extra precaution to clearly identify mock patients.)

2. At any drill, there must be at least 2 or 3 umpires who take no part in the drill itself; whose sole job it is to watch over and monitor the well-being of the mock patients. Being immobilized on a board may be extremely uncomfortable. People may suffer from tingling limbs; children in particular may have to go to the bathroom; and there is always the possibility that a real illness will arise. There may, as well, be some people who simply do not want to participate any longer. "Patients" must be able to communicate their needs and obtain immediate release for any of these problems. Of course any responder can and should do this—however, there should be umpires who will not wait to be asked, but will go about actively checking on the status of all "patients." At one drill we know of, which (as is usually the case) ran longer than expected, several "patients" were in danger of becoming hypothermic—a situation that was discovered by one of the responders almost by accident. Events of this sort must be carefully guarded against.

RADIO PRECAUTIONS

Because there is normally heavy radio traffic on the emergency frequencies, telephone all parties using them *before* running a drill to let them know where and when the drill will be held. They should be instructed that if they need to gain access to the frequency for a true emergency, they are to use the phrase, "*Breaker, true emergency*." From the time that call is heard there will be no more use of the radio for the drill until the real emergency is handled.

A secondary problem with radio communications is that strangers monitoring the frequency will hear the call for the MCI drill, and may think it is a real disaster. They may show up in their own vehicles, ready to offer help, but instead only creating confusion at the scene. To avoid this, use the word *mock* in the original call-up for the drill over all frequencies. Then, state that the incident is for training purposes and is *not* a genuine emergency.

PRECAUTIONS WITH VEHICLES

There are different schools of thought concerning the speed at which ambulances should travel during a drill. One school believes that more information and experience can be gained if ambulances travel at the speed they would use in a real emergency, and that they should use sirens and flashing lights. Our personal opinion is that the dangers inherent in this practice outweigh the rewards. We recommend that ambulances travel at nonemergency speeds.

There is also a danger that responders coming to the scene of the drill in their cars will be tempted to drive too fast. In our opinion, it should be made clear to everyone involved that daily speed limits and driving care are to be the rule. We feel that this will minimize the possibility of a mock responder becoming a true victim.

COVERING HOME BASES

With so much equipment and personnel taken off duty for drills, it is imperative that plans be made ahead of time to meet *all* normal EMS needs. True emergencies are as likely to happen during a drill as they are on any other day. Therefore, all units involved in the drill must make arrangements with other, noninvolved communites to cover their area for the normal, daily emergencies during the time when local personnel and equipment are tied up.

PSYCHOLOGICAL INFORMATION TO BE GAINED FROM DRILLS

Drills are learning experiences, but they can also be tools for evaluation of responders' emotional stability.

It is impossible to predict who will hold up well under the dreadful conditions to be found at a true MCI. It is generally true that those who tend to be overexcited and to do borderline work in daily EMS work will be worse at an MCI. However, it is *not* true that those who deal calmly with daily emergencies will therefore deal calmly with a Mass Casualty Incident. The conditions at an MCI are so nightmarish that even the steadiest-seeming person may lose some degree of control. You must assume that any responder may become emotionally unstable and ineffective during an MCI.

An MCI drill offers the opportunity to watch for signs of instability. Those who fall apart will bear close watching at a true incident.

Effective training is the key to avoiding or minimizing emotional instability. When everyone understands what his role is and why it is important to the plan as a whole, and when everyone has drilled enough to get some sense of the emotional nature of an MCI, personnel will have the feeling that they've done all this before. Thus, training and familiarity will tend to have a calming effect, promoting maximum efficiency in most responders.

Chapter 14

ALTERATIONS FOR WEATHER, LOCATION, AND SIZE

Modifying the General Plan

The general plan outlined in this text is just that—a *general* plan. It is designed to be a simple system that can serve as a basis for *any* MCI. By the same token, it must be adjusted and applied with unique detail to each *individual* MCI. Because all responders trained in the system will understand the common problems and needs, making necessary adjustments will be relatively easy and understandable to all involved.

Since no one can predetermine all of the possibilities or remember all of the potential alterations, no purpose would be served by detailing a wide range of specific incidents. Instead, through leadership and personnel well trained in a common system, these changes are effected incident-by-incident. Some examples will serve to illustrate the range of possibilities.

MODIFICATION EXAMPLE 1

Inclement weather conditions may make it inadvisable to have patients lying in the field. Two alternatives exist: either bring a sheltered environment to the field, or set up the collecting station in a nearby suitable environment. If 8 to 10 heated school buses can be brought to the field, boarded patients can be moved into the buses—which become the collecting station. Patients (except those in the Green category) can then be down-loaded from these "wards" into ambulances. In limited numbers, patients may even be transported in them.

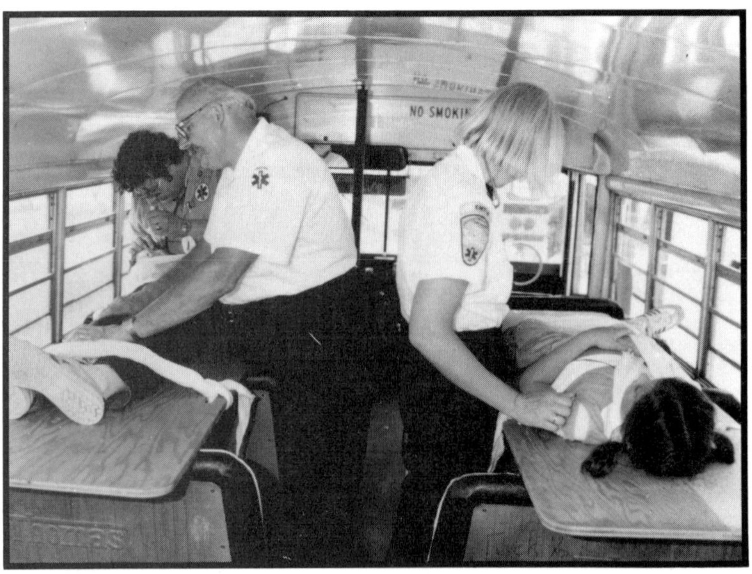

Another alternative is to take over 2 to 3 nearby residences (assuming no large, indoor heated space is immediate) to use as a patient collecting station. All furniture should be moved against the walls or outside, and only the ground floor should be employed.

A third alternative is to "haul and run" to the nearest school, hall, YMCA, supermarket, etc. Any place where there is indoor floor space for 60, 80, or more patients is suitable. Once the patients have been moved to this safe environment, they are assessed, triaged, and so on in accordance with the plan. Patients are then moved from this location to hospitals just as if this were the on-site collecting station.

It is important to note that an environment may be unsafe or hostile from causes other than weather. Terrorist activity, danger of ensuing explosion, imminent building collapse, or any other threatening condition at site may necessitate "haul and run" movement to a safe nearby location for stabilization and triage.

MODIFICATION EXAMPLE 2

If a plane crashes in a remote place only reachable on foot, then assessment, stabilization, and triage must occur at the site. However, special loading considerations now exist. The first deals with available porters to carry patients out; the second, with ambulance transport and hospital destination. A large number of strong porters should be amassed up the trail at the site, under the direction of one Transportation Officer. A second Transportation Officer will have to perform the usual "transport" function at the

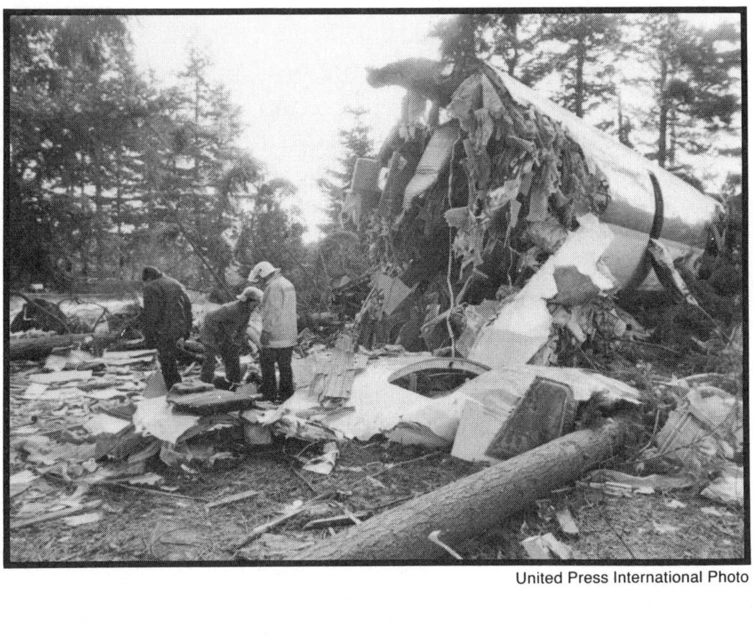

United Press International Photo

other end of the trail where the ambulances are waiting. Patients should be rapidly re-evaluated here and sent on as they arrive. A similar modification is necessary where patients must be moved from a pond by small boat, or by helicopter from a remote location.

MODIFICATION EXAMPLE 3

Incidents involving trains often have 2 fields of operation, one on each side of the train. Commonly, the train represents a barrier between these fields and it is often unrealistic to try to unify them. In this event it is better to divide the responders into groups according to need, and set up separate operations with separate collecting stations. Two sector Transport Officers, one at each collecting station, communicate with the senior Transport Officer who is placed at the first location common to leaving and arriving ambulances. He directs personnel to each side as needed. Note that all Red patients are moved from both sides before Yellow, and so on.

This type of split operation may also be necessary in large building collapses or structural fires.

MODIFICATION EXAMPLE 4

Ferry sinkings or any offshore MCIs usually produce survivors who are brought in by a large number of small craft. In these cases, a patient collecting station should be set up adjacent to a large dock or marina—for example, in the parking lot. The incident from dockside should operate as if it had occurred in the parking lot.

MODIFICATION EXAMPLE 5

When there are over 200 to 300 injured survivors of an MCI, unifying the response becomes a superhuman task. A more realistic approach is to bisect the incident in all ways—at the scene, in response call-up, and in the use of hospital facilities. Each sector operates as a separate disaster. For example, one Sub-Control Officer uses assets and directs transport to the north; another, to the south. Each sector takes care of about half the urgent patients. The overall Control Officer's job is limited to the more realistic tasks of adjusting patient spheres of activities to keep the operations balanced in overall urgency. The only other factors that are balanced are personnel and supplies.

The call-up pattern operates as if 2 disasters had occurred in nonadjacent communities—the actual one and one several towns away. Every plan should, therefore, include a second call-up to another nonadjacent community that will bring a full complement of 11 ambulances; EMTs; Control, Triage, and Transport Officers; and so on.

Conclusion

Variations and extensions of the general plan are as endless as the potential problems. They must be solved by on-site command personnel using field initiative, not by hundreds of alternative written plans. Command personnel must view each incident and adapt the general plan to fit it. Command personnel should participate in seminars at which hypothetical incidents are laid out. Then they can indicate how they would apply the general system to meet each incident's specific needs.

In spite of the immense variety of specific needs, one must remember that the more general needs and problems remain the same. They can be met in any community by realistic planning, by clear call-up and command systems, and by a commitment to include mass casualty in classroom training and drills as a meaningful part of training for *all* EMS personnel. The fact that 30, 60, or 80 victims have simultaneous needs does not lessen our responsibility to assure each patient of the care necessary for stabilization and of a fair chance for survival.

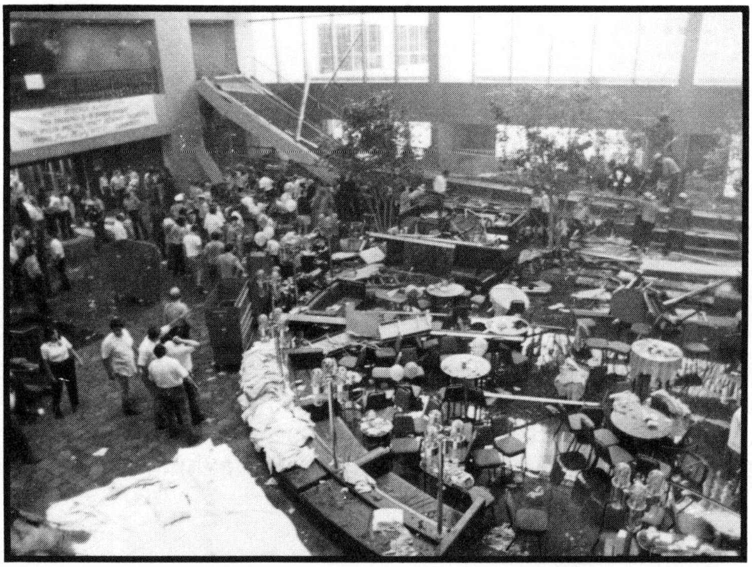

United Press International Photo

Index